THE DON'T SWEAT GUIDE
TO PREGNANCY

Other books by the editors of Don't Sweat Press

The Don't Sweat Affirmations
The Don't Sweat Guide for Couples
The Don't Sweat Guide for Graduates
The Don't Sweat Guide for Grandparents
The Don't Sweat Guide for Parents
The Don't Sweat Guide for Moms
The Don't Sweat Guide for Weddings
The Don't Sweat Guide to Golf
The Don't Sweat Stories
The Don't Sweat Guide to Travel
The Don't Sweat Guide to Weight Loss
The Don't Sweat Guide to Taxes
The Don't Sweat Guide for Dads
The Don't Sweat Guide to Retirement
The Don't Sweat Guide for Teachers
The Don't Sweat Guide for Newlyweds
The Don't Sweat Guide to Cooking
The Don't Sweat Guide to Your New Home
The Don't Sweat Guide to Holidays
The Don't Sweat Guide to Entertaining
The Don't Sweat Guide to Your Job Search
The Don't Sweat Guide to Your Finances

THE DON'T SWEAT GUIDE
TO PREGNANCY

Making the Most of the Months
Before the Baby

By the Editors of Don't Sweat Press
Foreword by Richard Carlson, Ph.D.,
and Kristine Carlson

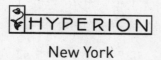

New York

ISBN: 1-4013-0761-2

Hyperion books are available for special promotions and premiums.
For details contact Michael Rentas, Manager, Inventory and Premium Sales,
Hyperion, 77 West 66th Street, 11th floor, New York, New York 10023,
or call 212-456-0133.

FIRST EDITION

10 9 8 7 6 5 4 3 2 1

Contents

Foreword

I have to admit that when I was asked to write the foreword to this book, the first thing I did was run to Kris and ask for her help! Being a father, I was able to experience Kris's pregnancies vicariously, of course, but obviously, it's not the same as going through it yourself. So this foreword is a joint creation from the two of us.

We'd estimate that ninety-five percent of the women we know have told us that pregnancy was, simultaneously, the most stressful and the most wonderful experience that they have ever gone through. Although a few would not repeat it, no one that we know has ever said to either one of us that they would rather not have gone through it. That's pretty amazing, when you think about it.

The editors of Don't Sweat Press have done a beautiful job of reminding all of us what a miracle it is to have a baby. Without denying the real-life burdens or the physical discomfort of pregnancy, the editors have emphasized the beauty, grace, magic, and miracle of birth.

Whether you are considering having a baby, are currently pregnant, or have just gone through the process, this book is a must-read. It is inspiring, hopeful, practical, and filled with creative ideas to get you through the process in the least stressful way possible.

There's no question that pregnancy is stressful on the mother, both physically and emotionally. It takes its toll. The editors of this book have found a very gentle way to address that stress in a non-lecturing, non-threatening way that speaks to the needs of women during this important time of life.

If you or someone that you care about is going through a pregnancy, this is an ideal book for her to keep at her side. It's a comfort that can be turned to in good times and bad for a burst of wisdom, a hint of insight, or a creative solution.

We both wish that this book would have been available when we had our two children, because we would have referred to it often. We do know, however, that many of our friends will be receiving it as a gift in the years to come. We hope and pray that if you or someone you love is pregnant, either now or in the future, both the mother and child are happy and healthy! We send you our love.

Richard and Kristine Carlson
Benicia, California, 2004

THE DON'T SWEAT GUIDE
TO PREGNANCY

1.
Waiting and Wishing

Perhaps you've bought this book in anticipation of conception. Anticipation can be the most exciting part of any event. Indeed, pregnancy itself is nine months of anticipating that little angel that you will someday cradle in your arms. Maybe a girlfriend gave you the book because it was her own favorite pregnancy book. She knows that you and your loved one are hoping to conceive. In fact, it may seem that everyone knows what the two of you are doing behind closed doors.

Suddenly, your intimate moments with your mate have become conception marathons. Instead of enjoying your romantic times together, you're juggling duty with stopwatches and ovulation kits. At some point, many couples quit answering the phones when their married friends call to ask, "Any news yet?"

Each month the stakes for fertilization get higher. You may swear that you feel nausea and cravings—and then you're disappointed. You and your partner may start to worry that something is wrong. Most often the answer is that you are trying too hard.

Here are the facts. Eighty-five percent of couples trying to conceive are successful within a year. While some women need only to think about conception for it to occur, most of us need a little bit longer.

Professionals recommend that a couple contact a physician for potential problems only after they have tried to conceive for one year. (The exception is women over thirty-five. They should call their doctors after six months, since time may be of the essence if there is a need to correct a physical problem.)

So relax! You have a year. Continue your healthy lifestyle. Tell your married friends that you've decided to wait a while before you have a baby. Make dates with your partner and actually enjoy your intimate relations again.

After all, every woman has heard a story of a couple that finally conceived once they quit trying. Why not quit trying for a while and put some fun back into your fun? Who knows what might happen?

2.

Share the Joyous News

You will always be able to recall the exact moment that you learned you were pregnant. For many, the moment happened when they stared, blurry-eyed, at the stick from a drugstore pregnancy kit. Thinking back, they may smile fondly when they remember that morning of awe and excitement.

Why not also create a special moment for the other person who will be the most important in your child's life? Perhaps you and your loved one can take the test together. If that's not the case, take care in how you break the news to him. You could e-mail him while he's at work or you could set the stage for a romantic moment that will be a delicious memory etched in his heart for years to come.

Perhaps you could give him a gift that hints at his impending parenthood, such as a book of baby names. Tuck a Father's Day card into his briefcase. Maybe even break the news to him at a restaurant when he asks why you're drinking milk instead of wine.

However you decide to let him know that he will soon be a new father, take a few moments to rejoice in the news together. Give both of you a memory to cherish eighty years down the road.

3.

Savor the Secret

It is important for a woman to tell her partner about the new life growing inside of her. After all, the father-to-be will also need a full nine months to adjust to the idea of parenthood. Besides, how else is she going to explain all of the time that she spends in the bathroom?

However, it's not necessary to tell everyone right away. Why not allow yourselves a few days or weeks to savor a delicious secret?

Some couples wait until after the first trimester to announce their pregnancy. That is when the highest risk of miscarriage is past. Many couples, however, want to share the wonderful news with their friends and family immediately. After all, isn't that what friends are for? In fact, you might go crazy waiting until you've broken the news to your partner so that you can tell your best friend.

Best friends and mothers aside, why not savor the secret for a little while? Word will spread. In the meantime, when you wink to your honey across a crowded room, it will be that much more delightful if the crowd doesn't know that you're carrying a secret.

4.

Explore All of Your Emotions

Of course, you're thrilled to be pregnant—or perhaps you are not. Your opinion of this whole baby thing may even change from one moment to the next. Whether this was or was not a planned pregnancy, you will go through a multitude of emotions—and they are all perfectly normal.

When you feel good about being pregnant, revel in the loving feeling of growing your darling little baby inside your body. Allow yourself to picture your little one running around the house wearing nothing but a diaper. Immerse yourself in your nurturing side when it takes over.

It is just as important to allow yourself to feel a little worried and a little nervous about the biggest lifestyle change that you will ever experience. Notice that the operative words here are "a little." Of course, you will feel a little worried and nervous. That's the first sign that you are going to be a wonderful parent. No one actually knows how to raise a child. We just do our best and hope for the best.

You might even be a little angry when you can't make it through the morning without losing your breakfast, or concerned that you are not where you thought you would be financially when you started a family. (Only about one in a hundred families are financially set before they have a child. If you had waited until you felt you were completely ready, you may never have had kids.)

Allow yourself to grieve for your current lifestyle. Understand that everyone feels nervous about raising children. Even those old veterans who have raised several of them will tell you that there are no hard and fast rules. Recognize your frustration with your pregnancy symptoms or financial fears. Respect your emotions. Then let them go, and move on.

The pendulum of emotions swings for all pregnant women. Soon enough, you will be overjoyed when the baby kicks against your tummy or when you spot a little hat that will be adorable on a newborn. Just ride your emotions back up to the crest of the wave.

5.

Believe in Your Doctor

For the next nine months, you will find that your priorities fall this way: Your baby is the most important thing in the world. You, and your health, will place second. Unless your partner is a doctor, he will probably rank in a third-place tie with your obstetrician/gynecologist (OB/GYN).

An obstetrician is a doctor who focuses on pregnant women and delivers their babies. The gynecologist is the doctor of women's health who has been prescribing your birth control pills for years. The same doctor makes the switch from birth prevention to birth preparation when the stick turns blue.

It is imperative to examine your relationship with your current doctor. Do you believe that your doctor is competent? This is most important. If you question your doctor's abilities, you will not be able to trust him or her throughout your pregnancy—and trust becomes paramount in pregnancy. If your doctor tells you to get off your feet for three days or to give up your diet sodas, you need to believe that he or she means it, and that there is a reason for it.

Does your doctor listen to you? Does your doctor make the time to talk to you? With all of the insurance paperwork and restrictions that some doctors face, they may feel overwhelmed by their patient load and not take the time to talk to their patients. Such a doctor is not the one for you during your pregnancy. Pregnant women have a lot of questions. Look for a doctor who encourages interaction and communication. Would you feel comfortable calling your doctor on a Sunday afternoon if you have an emergency?

If you want to find a new doctor, or a midwife, start by canvassing your girlfriends about their own OB/GYNs. A good referral speaks volumes about a doctor's standing. In your initial consultation with a new caregiver, make sure that you address issues that are important to you. For instance, if you want an all-natural birth in a pool of water, your obstetrician had better be aware of it. If you plan to take painkillers from the moment that you walk through the hospital doors, be sure that your doctor recommends that for you.

Finding a doctor who makes you feel comfortable will be the best thing that you can do for yourself throughout your pregnancy. You'll worry a little less about your baby and yourself, and that will even make your partner happier—even if he does have to share third place with your OB/GYN.

6.

Allow Friends and Family to Help

By now, it has become an old saying: "It takes a village to raise a child." If this is your first child, you will learn that there is much truth to that statement—and it starts when the child is still in the womb.

As women, we try to do it all. Not only do we want to do it all, we want to do it all now, and we want to prove that we can do it all by ourselves without any help. Why? Why is it so difficult for us to accept help? We often believe that those who are offering their assistance are "only being nice," and if we accept their invitations, then we are actually "imposing" on them.

Nothing could be further from the truth. Our friends and family want to help us. They want to be involved in the magical journey called pregnancy. When your best friend says, "Please call if you need anything," she is actually saying, "This is great. I want to share this experience with you. Please let me do that."

The next time that someone offers to help, let him or her do so. Try saying "Great! Could you watch my other kids on Saturday while I take a nap?" Why not let your mother-in-law know that you would love it if she could pick up your dry cleaning the next time she is going out that way? Give your best friend a "gift" by hinting that this would be the ideal time for that dinner invitation that she's mentioned, to save yourself some kitchen duty.

Don't forget to let the daddy-to-be sort some laundry while you relax with your feet elevated. If he offers (or you hint), let it happen. Do not be upset when he mixes your grays with yellows. Be thankful for the rest so that you can tackle your other responsibilities.

It takes a village to raise a child—and they want to help. Who are you to argue?

7.

Celebrate Your (Growing) Body

Marilyn Monroe. Raquel Welch. Sophia Loren. Each is considered to be an icon of feminine beauty—and not a single one of them wore a size two dress.

What exactly is it that makes these women so dazzling? Perhaps it's their full busts—or maybe their curvaceous hips. Don't forget about that thick, shiny hair.

Does any of this sound familiar? Have you looked in a mirror lately? Your bust is fuller. Your hips are curvaceous. You have shiny hair. You have it all.

You…are…gorgeous.

Yes, it is difficult for us to believe that bigger can be more beautiful. After all, we live in a world where women are considered beautiful only if clothes are falling off them. The thought of gaining back those five holiday pounds that we finally lost can be mortifying. You don't even want to dwell on the thirty to forty pounds that pregnancy has to offer.

Before you swear off chocolate for life—or, at least, until the next craving—remember that much of the weight will drop off quickly after the birth. Until then, enjoy your growing body. You have, no doubt, heard people say that there is nothing more beautiful than a pregnant woman. They mean what they say—and it is not purely an intellectual observation. Several studies have suggested that pregnant women truly are more attractive to the human eye, because they epitomize the qualities that we equate with femininity—fuller busts, lips, and hair.

So embrace your growing body. Swing those hips. Flip that hair. Of course, your middle will be a bit thicker, but who will notice when the rest of you looks so fabulous?

8.

Understand Daddy's Fears

You're pregnant, and of course, you're a little nervous. You have a new life growing inside of you. Your own life is changing day by day. Soon, you will be a mother—with all those responsibilities that go with the job.

Sometimes, it seems that the father-to-be is just not as understanding as he should be—or is it possible that we mothers-to-be are just not as understanding as we could be? Dads do, after all, have fears of their own. Although most men are reluctant to discuss their feelings, that doesn't mean their concerns don't exist.

First of all, let's remember that society places the financial burden of child rearing on the man's shoulders. Unbeknownst to you, your partner may be awake all night long, worried about providing food, shelter, and clothing for his newborn. It can be terrifying to know that someone depends on you so completely.

Then there is the fear of not being a good father. More accurately, he may worry that he will not be "as good as his father," or, sadly, that he will turn out to be just like his own father.

However, most of his fears may center on you. Soon, he will no longer be the most important person in your life. That can sting. Scarier still is the thought that something harmful might happen to you during pregnancy and childbirth. It's already a given that you will experience some discomfort along the way. There is not a single thing that your man can do except to watch his beloved suffer. Imagine how that must feel. He also knows that there are risks (albeit very, very slight risks) associated with childbirth. How could he ever forgive himself if something happened to you because you carried his child?

Although his concerns may seem a little silly to you (which is why he doesn't voice them), your dismay that your jeans no longer fit may feel somewhat trivial to him. If he seems a little preoccupied, that's because he is.

Okay, so he gets to skip the morning sickness and stretch marks—but that doesn't mean that he's not being affected by the pregnancy. In fact, he may be thinking about it constantly—and be just as nervous as you are.

9.

Accept Your Limitations

Your best friend brags that she competed in a 10K run in her fourth month of pregnancy. Good for her. Did she mention that she was nineteen years old and walked to the point that her mother picked her up in the car—around the four-kilometer marker?

Your mother-in-law tells about the day that she was sailing across the Atlantic and went into labor. She probably doesn't talk about the team of doctors on board the ship and the very effective sedative that they administered.

Forget the bragging. The women who tell these stories were just as exhausted as you are. They slept in on the weekends. They slowed down their activities. They spent several hours reading, just like you do.

Right now, your body must come first, and your body needs rest. That is what it has been trying to tell you. It's okay if you skip one—or several—block party meetings. No one will be offended if you miss your turn to host the book club. Your bedroom really doesn't need to be scrubbed down every other weekend. Most people understand the strains of pregnancy.

Remember, you're just a little busy right now growing another human being inside of you. Maybe you should stop for a moment and consider where, exactly, you should be devoting your energy. After all, your pregnant body is tired for a reason. It's telling you to slow down, because it has work to do!

10.

Look Absolutely Fabulous

This isn't your mother's pregnancy—and many thanks for that. No offense, Mom. Tent dresses with red polka dots and ruffled necklines looked splendid on you, but fashion has changed. Today's mom-to-be doesn't hide her baby-to-be under yards of fabric. Instead, she looks radiant by featuring the beauty of the life growing within her. Fitted clothes celebrate a pregnancy rather than disguising it.

Modern maternity clothes are worth the trip to the mall. Besides, what better excuse could there be for a woman to buy clothes than pregnancy? Still, being stylish can be a challenge, not to mention expensive, when one's dress size changes week by week.

As tempting as it may be to run out for a new wardrobe the moment that you know you are pregnant, why not relax and wear your stretchy clothes for a little while until you figure out what you really need? Is your wardrobe mostly based on your work attire? Dinner outfits? Casual wear?

Your new-mother friends will still have half of their closets dedicated to maternity garments. These clothes tend to make the rounds among girlfriends. Soon after you announce your pregnancy, your doorbell will ring. The items that get traded the most are the ones that are the most useful. They are:

- Overalls—They are the weekend pregnancy uniform. Wear a colorful top underneath to let your bosom upstage your belly.

- Leggings—They go great with cropped tops, snug sweaters, and a man's button-down shirt.

- Light cotton or knit dresses—They're sleek and feminine, and they grow with you. Dresses that tie in the back have the long haul advantage.

- Little black dress—Pregnant or not, where would any woman be without one?

Borrow what you can. Buy what you need. Wear the outfits with grace. Then pass them on when you're finished. Who knows when they might just make the rounds back to your closet?

11.

Honor Your Body

There will be times that your body will feel alien to you. You may wonder: Whose body is this? Why don't I like pastrami anymore? Am I really craving peanut butter? I haven't had that in years! Why does everything feel so strange?

For most of your life, you've taken the lead with your body. You've decided when to eat, as well as what to eat. You've chosen when to nap, when to exercise, and when to take an aspirin. Now, suddenly, your body is taking over. It's telling you that it's hungry. That's called morning sickness. You may have skipped breakfast for the last twenty years, but now your stomach wants breakfast—and it wants it immediately!

Your body is also—obviously—very tired. It doesn't matter that you've never gone to bed before midnight. Your body now wants to turn in when it starts to grow dark. "Forget the chores," your aching limbs tell you. "Let's go to sleep."

You may be tempted to try a mind-over-matter approach, willing your stomach to be quiet and your legs to keep going. You might even consider administering a quick fix, like a cup of coffee—but why? Right now your body is performing an amazing feat—a feat that it was meant to perform—the creation of life. That's no small task for you or your body.

Your body knows exactly what it is doing. Of course, you're hungry. Your body needs extra calories to grow a new life inside of it. Of course, you're tired. It takes a lot of energy to grow a baby. With all due respect, your body knows this drill better than you do—that's its job.

Even if you can't believe that you have a reason to be hungry or tired, your body knows better. Try eating a peanut butter and pickle sandwich, if that's what your body wants. Take a nap (if you can) when your eyelids start to droop. You may be surprised at how much you like it.

Trust that your body knows what is best right now. Listen closely, and honor your body's requests.

12.

Delight in All That Food

Perhaps you are naturally thin and cannot seem to gain weight. If so, you're a lucky girl. Now turn the page and leave the rest of us alone.

For most of us, this will be the first time (since the age of twelve, when we discovered body image) that we can eat without guilt. Yahoo!

One pregnant woman actually admitted to sitting cross-legged on the floor in front of her open refrigerator. When her husband walked in, she had a fork in her right hand while she juggled three containers of leftover food in her left. She reasoned that anything within fork reach—over her belly—was fair game.

Another woman bearing a child refused to leave the house without two sliced apples and a sleeve of whole wheat crackers in her purse. She even took her favorite snack with her when she was going out to eat. Another woman used pregnancy as an opportunity to become somewhat of an expert on chocolate truffles.

Eat away and enjoy!

In fact, why not make the very most of the situation? Take a cooking class. That will help to cure both your physical cravings and your emotional yearnings to nest. No time for a cooking class? Grab your favorite cookbook, and try some of those recipes that you've always wanted to make. After all, so what if you eat a second helping of potatoes? Remember that your body needs extra calories right now.

Also remember to make nutrition a primary consideration. Why grab the Cheez Doodles when the block of cheddar has more calcium? Reach for the beans—full of protein and folates (ultra-important B vitamins essential for cell growth and brain development)—instead of the processed crackers. We all know how much better for you yogurt is over ice cream.

Still, unless your doctor has suggested that you need to watch your caloric intake, the weight that you gain should be the absolute least of your worries. Until then, eat nutritiously, and skip the guilt.

13.

Please Feed Me Right

"*I'm hungry!*" screams the cry from within. Your stomach begins to twitch with a low rumble, which quickly grows into a somersault-type roar. You start to feel a little lightheaded. Oops, you're dizzy. It's time to sit down.

This can happen at the most inconvenient times. While you're discussing the agenda for next Monday's business meeting with your staff, your vision blurs a little bit. All you can think about are jelly-filled donuts!

When you're pregnant, your body will sometimes demand that you drop everything now—right now—for some food. Before running off to the closest vending machine, stop and listen—really listen—to exactly what your body wants. Your natural instinct may be to grab some peanut butter crackers to satisfy your hunger. While you could certainly eat a worse snack than peanut butter crackers, they might not be satisfying your baby's hunger as well as you might think.

There are certain things that your body needs during pregnancy. Those extra 300 or so calories a day that your body demands do carry a nutritional price tag. Be sure to balance your diet with dairy products for calcium, grains and vegetables for fiber, and dark leafy greens for folates.

Experts suggest that you follow these basics:

- Nine or more servings of breads, cereals, and grains (at least four should be whole grain)
- Seven or more servings of fruits and vegetables
- Three or more servings of milk and milk products
- Three or more servings of protein, such as lean meat, poultry, fish, eggs, nuts, and dried beans

Also be sure to quench your thirst. Fluids help your body process nutrients. Without enough fluids, you may start to feel sluggish and constipated. Aim for at least six to eight glasses of fluid a day. Water is optimal, but juice, milk, and herbal teas can also help to satisfy your body's growing needs.

For full menus or snack ideas, there are several quality books on the market and web pages on the Internet, for nutrition during pregnancy. When your belly roars, be sure to satisfy it with the nutritional content that it really wants.

14.

Before You Knew

After the initial excitement of discovering a pregnancy, many women's thoughts turn to concern about the things that they may have done before they discovered the news. Ideally, a woman of childbearing age who intends to get pregnant will have taken precautions to guard her health. It is now common knowledge that a woman who is considering pregnancy or trying to conceive should take prenatal vitamins, eat nutritiously, and abstain from alcohol, tobacco, and potentially dangerous behavior.

Having said that, not every situation is ideal, not every pregnancy is planned, and not a single one of us is perfect. What if you indulged in a glass of wine before you found out that you were pregnant? Perhaps you exercised strenuously last week. Maybe you recently survived the death of a loved one and have concerns about the emotional effects on your unborn baby.

However, the first trimester is the most crucial to the development of a baby. Right?

Yes, but take this into consideration: As you know, the sperm fertilizes the egg. The egg spends the next two weeks traveling down the fallopian tubes and free-floating in the uterus. At this point, the egg is called a zygote and is little more than a lump of cells. The zygote is extremely protected.

The egg then implants itself into the wall of the womb. If there is no implantation, a woman sheds the lining of her uterus and menstruates. If the egg does attach itself, it becomes an embryo, and you are officially pregnant.

This is not to say that the zygote is protected from everything. It is imperative that you discuss any concerns—from prescription medications to that 10K race you just ran—with your doctor. For the most part, however, don't obsess over your behavior in the very early days of the pregnancy. Your baby will probably be just fine. Take extra precautions now to protect him or her throughout the next nine months.

15.

Take Care of Your Aches and Pains

In the beginning of a pregnancy, your body temperature will increase, producing a mild fever. You'll be tired. Your breasts will be sore, and you may have cramps. Some women even experience swelling, indigestion, headaches, and difficulty breathing. Sounds like fun, huh? Yet it's all very short-lived.

Your doctor will give you a list of the symptoms to call about. Certainly, if you have a pressing question—or if you have a nagging feeling that "something just isn't right"—pick up the phone and call your doctor. However, if your question is, "Do all pregnant women feel like this?" the answer is probably yes. It's achy. It's tiring. It's emotional. And it's wonderful.

These are simply the pains of pregnancy. They will get worse toward the end, but they will be soon forgotten after the fact. For now, the best thing that you can do is to make yourself comfortable.

Ask your friends what they did to alleviate their aches and pains. Many women swear on wearing a bra to bed for support and lying flat on a heating pad to relieve tired backs. Others could not have made it if they hadn't elevated their feet at every given opportunity. Some ate antacids. Although physicians warn against taking aspirin during pregnancy, as it thins the blood, many do allow acetaminophen. (Check with your own doctor first.)

The most important way to treat your aching body may be simple common sense. Why eat that burrito when you know that it will haunt you? Stay off your feet whenever you can to ease those ankles. Put down the laundry basket when your back hurts. Give yourself a break, and take care of those aches and pains.

16.

Take This Opportunity to Put You First

If this is your first child, then you are going to be in utter shock at how much another human being will depend on you for survival. This is not meant to scare you. You will adore the time that you spend nurturing that sweet little angel. However, soon you may spend every waking moment doing so. Right now, your body is very devoted to creating this amazing being. That means that you need to choose where you put your energy. Why not (probably for the first time in your life) put yourself first?

Do you really need to host your gardening club at your house over the next nine months? Can someone else host the meetings? Is that volunteer work taking too much time? Why not scale back your duties? What about all of those errands? Can you find a dry cleaner that delivers, or share the grocery shopping with your partner?

You're pregnant. People will understand. In fact, they will probably expect this sort of thing from you.

Put that energy into doing things that you've wanted to do for yourself. Bring the photo album up to date. Redecorate the living room—just remember to ask a girlfriend with a toddler for advice on that one. Childproofing has a way of taking over a house. Why not make it baby-friendly to begin with? Maybe you've wanted to learn Spanish or play the piano. Do it now—while your unborn baby can hear you. After all, babies can hear in the womb.

Take some time out for yourself while you still can. Soon, your days (and your heart) will belong to the most beautiful little creature in the world, but for now, you have a little free time and a great excuse to put yourself first.

17.

Morning Sick, All Day Sick

Some women skip merrily through their pregnancies without a hint of nausea. Others spend the first three months with their heads in the toilet. Most of us fall somewhere in between the two extremes. In fact, fifty to eighty percent of all pregnant women experience morning sickness.

Morning sickness is a misnomer. It can strike any time of day or night. The cause is simply a tidal wave of progesterone flooding through your body. The cure is—well, there is no cure. If there were, no pregnant lady would ever turn green at the sight of raspberries again.

Raspberries—you used to love them. Now, a mere whiff and you feel nauseated. Ditto for garlic, coffee, and toothpaste. Food aversions may be your first line of defense against morning sickness. If you can identify and stay away from the scents that affect your tummy, you may avoid the impending queasiness. By contrast, foods that you are craving may actually help to calm the churning seas of the stomach.

In addition to listening to your body's cues, there are several other things you can do to help alleviate these particular symptoms.

- Eat several small meals throughout the day.
- Drink more water. Dehydration can cause morning sickness.
- Carry saltines or other bland snacks with you to help curb nausea.
- Try ginger—tea, candies, or capsules.
- Take your prenatal vitamins on a full stomach or before bed.
- Try acupressure bands for seasickness. They're noninvasive, drug free, and work for many women.
- Avoid belts and tight waistbands.

If none of this works, you may want to talk to your doctor regarding other suggestions and options. In general, most expectant women simply learn to grab a sick bag and move on with their day.

The good news is that morning sickness almost always disappears after the third month. One day, you're running to every bathroom you see. The next morning, you wake up hungry instead of nauseated, and you've never felt better. You'll still run to the bathroom, but now it will be due to the call of your bladder instead of the scream of your stomach.

18.
Laugh Off Those Embarrassing Moments

Every woman who has ever been pregnant has an embarrassing story to tell about her baby-carrying days. After all, mommies-to-be are no longer in complete control of their bodies, and their babies aren't really interested in social appearances. If they think that it's time to let a little air out to create some more room inside the belly, then it's time to do that. Never mind the fact that you're standing in a quiet crowded elevator. It's time to pass the gas, Mom, okay?

Another place that babies like to make themselves known is at the supermarket. For some reason, many mommies recall leaving their carts to race to the restroom before they tossed cookies on the—well, the cookie display. A few have suffered the indignity of laughing so hard at a dinner party that they lost control of their bladders. Others have turned green at the sight of the hostess's famous ham soufflé.

There's no use worrying about whether or not an embarrassing moment might happen to you while you're pregnant. It will. It's all part of the charm of pregnancy. Besides, every woman needs to have an embarrassing pregnancy story to tell to her Lamaze friends. When these embarrassing moments happen, just smile sweetly and say, "I'm pregnant."

Chances are that the people in the elevator, in the supermarket, or at the dinner party have their own embarrassing tales, or they know someone who does. They know that bodily functions are sometimes beyond your control. If they didn't already know that, they've just gained valuable knowledge for the future.

19.

Keep Things in Perspective

Welcome to your initiation into the sorority of motherhood. Please do not let it scare you.

Yes, from now until you give birth, most women that you meet will insist on reciting their terrible labor stories. Every mother has one. Bear in mind that many of the stories are quite exaggerated. Considering their contractions and the intensity of the situation, some may have embellished a few of the details here and there. It certainly sounds more courageous to have been in labor for twenty-four hours than for three hours, doesn't it?

Don't let the tall tales shake you. You may well have your own "I was in labor for eighteen hours" story, even though you might not even realize that you're in labor and keep shopping through the first five hours of the whole ordeal.

While pregnant, you may also encounter the "alarmists." These are your otherwise upbeat friends and coworkers who will be quite concerned when they caution that you look pale. Maybe you should rest. Perhaps you shouldn't lift anything. Some will tell you this every day of your pregnancy until you give birth to a beautifully healthy ten-pound baby.

Also, medical science from here on in will state that everything you do is bad for you and your unborn child. When you're pregnant, a new study regarding the health of unborn children will seem to pop up every day. Do not ignore the reports that you see. It is, however, a good idea to read the report fully. While the magic of medical science has brought us to the point of very, very few birth defects, far too many studies are published prior to a conclusive result. The headline that reads "Exposure to Wood May be Harmful to Human Fetuses" could actually turn out to be a story that states, "Pregnant women who breathe sawdust 365 days a year might possibly be putting their children at risk. The results are inconclusive."

Additionally, try not to fret about the results of every test your caregiver administers. With all of the tests today, we are more aware than ever of the complications that can beset our babies. In fact, statistics can illustrate for us that many more healthy babies are born each year than babies with birth defects.

New mothers are already at risk for conjuring up the worst-case scenarios for their babies. Our friends and the media may not help. Every pregnant lady has her concerns. The point is to try to keep it all in perspective.

20.

Enjoy Your Dreams

One of the best parts of pregnancy can be the increased dream activity. One of the worst parts of pregnancy can be the increased dream activity.

Experts believe that a pregnant woman's increased progesterone level may contribute to more frequent and vivid dreams. They also agree that restless sleep has a lot to do with it. With a changing body and a squirming baby in one's belly, we tend to awaken more during the night than usual. This keeps us in a light stage of sleep, referred to as REM (Rapid Eye Movement) sleep, for longer periods of time. REM sleep is the stage in which most of our dreaming is done. So not only are you in a stage of dream sleep more often, but you are awakened from that state more frequently, and therefore, you have a greater chance of remembering your dreams.

In general, dreams are fun. They're like discovering a part of yourself that you didn't know existed. Many women have reported having incredibly physical dreams while they were pregnant.

While the fun dreams can be intoxicating and make you want to sleep more, other dreams truly can be nightmares. At some time or another, you might dream that you left your baby on the hood of your car and drove off. You may have vivid images of giving birth to a kitten. You may even have a vision that a darling daughter is finally born—and she looks just like your uncle, mustache and all.

It is reported that the most common dreams among pregnant women are images of water, talking animals, romance, and large buildings. While dream psychologists often differ on what the meaning of all these things are, one thing is for certain. Your dreams will interrupt your sleep!

Enjoy the fun dreams. Let go of the annoying ones. They are not visions of things to come. They are the same silly dreams that belong to all pregnant women. Shake it off. Go back to sleep.

21.

Expect Mood Swings

Your defense? You're pregnant. Your crime? Mood swings. Most women have experienced a small amount of premenstrual syndrome (PMS). One minute, you're calm and collected. The next, you're snapping at your hairdresser for wearing an orange smock. Those same hormones that cause the PMS roller coaster are now flooding through your body in record force. Your emotional pendulum is working overtime.

Many mothers-to-be find themselves utterly depressed if they read a news story about an infant's death. Most suddenly weep with joy during a diaper commercial that they've seen a hundred times before. Others may dedicate a popular song on the radio to their unborn child. From the minute that the song captures their heart, these women are sure to shed a tear whenever the song is played— whether they are alone in the car or standing in a crowd of coworkers at the local deli.

The good news about mood swings is that they are expected. There is not a single woman who can claim an even temperament during her pregnancy. The bad news is that you probably feel somewhat crazy, and your friends and family can verify that you are—that is, if you can find them. As supportive as your loved ones want to be, you may be a little difficult to be around right now. People aren't sure what to expect. They've spent years getting to know you, and now they don't know you at all. Sometimes, you don't even know yourself.

Yes, you are probably a little moodier than usual, even if you don't necessarily see it. When you catch yourself getting worked up about something, stop. Are these the hormones talking? Is this really an issue that you'll care about tomorrow? Where have your friends and family run off to this time? Perhaps a cup of tea and a warm bath might just be in order.

When the sight of a cute puppy or smudged nail polish makes you weep for a good half-hour, you're probably just experiencing those pregnancy mood swings. It's all part of the process. It will only last for a few more months. Until then, just try to remember that you are, after all, pregnant, and you might just be a little moody at times.

22.

Calmly Make the Announcement

Some of your friends and coworkers may have already guessed your status before you make the big announcement. It's the little things that give you away—ordering milk at lunch instead of your usual red wine, or taking your daily vitamins in the ladies' room.

Some will see the connection to your recent behavior like the flick of a switch. "Ah-ha! So that's why you've been eating a dozen donuts for breakfast every morning." Others will be taken completely by surprise. "Wow!" is about all that they will say.

All of them will be full of questions. Was this planned? How does your partner feel about it? Do you want a boy or a girl? What names do you have picked out? When is it due? Are you going to breastfeed or bottle-feed? Will you go back to work?

Guess what—you don't have to give them all of the answers to the questions. Chances are that you don't even know all of the answers to these questions yet. Some of the inquiries may even feel intrusive. Often, we keep our personal and professional lives separate.

Are these appropriate topics to discuss with coworkers? Engaging in this type of discussion may make you feel as if you've compromised your professionalism.

If you feel comfortable discussing the details, enjoy the chatter. If, however, you have no preference between a boy and a girl, or you simply would rather not talk about the matter, be up front (yet polite) with your friends. A simple "I honestly don't know" or "That's really a private matter" will get the point across without making anyone uncomfortable.

You may also choose to inject a little humor into the situation. When the people in your carpool want to know, "How does your husband feel about your pregnancy?" why not counter with a quick, "I'll let you know once I tell him." Just make sure that they know you're kidding. You know how hard it is to stop office rumors once they start.

23.

Take Control of Your Memory

There may come a day when you're driving home from work and you forget to turn down the same street that you have driven down for five years now. There may also come a time when you drive all the way to the mall to return a sweater, only to realize that you didn't bring the sweater—and you're at the wrong mall. You may even wake up one morning and realize that you've forgotten your own mother's phone number.

No, this is not the beginning of senility. This is simply the distracted state provided by all good pregnancies. Everything may seem a bit hazy, foggy, or disconnected. On top of the physical effects are your own preoccupied thoughts: "Where *is* the closest bathroom, anyway?"

It is said that pregnancy insomnia prepares one for life with a newborn. So does this temporary state of confusion. Soon, life will revolve around the 389 things to do every day for baby. A little organization can go a long way.

Why not make things easier for yourself in the long run by starting now? Get in the habit of putting your keys in the same spot every day. Write down conversations with your coworkers. If you're not already a chronic list-maker, at least jot down a quick morning "to-do" list. When all else fails, don't hesitate to remind people that you're pregnant. "What was that you mentioned about a meeting on Tuesday? Pregnancy plays with one's memory."

Taking a few steps now to ensure smooth sailing may prevent a lot of wasted time and frustration down the road. Sure, there will still be the time that you show up at your in-laws' house only to realize that you forgot your father-in-law's first name—but at least you found your keys and turned down the right street to get to the house!

24.

A Less-Than-Enthusiastic Response

Uh-oh. The baby's father isn't doing cartwheels. Or maybe it's your mother, his mother, or your college roommate who seems to be less than overjoyed about your pregnancy. People may seem less than excited for a variety of reasons.

Before you allow yourself to become overemotional about the situation (something that pregnant women often do), take a step back, and then take a deep breath. Allow the person with whom you are sharing the news to do the same.

The baby thing might simply need some time to sink in. Your baby's father, for instance, may be in the midst of a stressful job predicament. Until he can settle that situation, he may not be able to deal with the fact that he's about to become a father. To you, he may not seem very excited. In truth, he may be keeping his emotions in check until he has the time to deal with them appropriately.

Your elders may not seem to be too happy, either. Again, give them time to absorb the information. They may wonder if you are ready to become a parent. Then they'll remember that their own parents wondered if they were ready to become parents, and they did just fine.

Other special people in your life may feel that they're going to lose you, and in a way, they are. The simple facts are that you won't have as much in common with your childless friends, and you won't have as much time to dedicate to them, either. Soon, they will discover that they're not losing a friend, they're gaining a baby, and watching a newborn grow and develop is one of the most magical experiences of all.

Respect that other people in your life also need to adjust to the news of your pregnancy. Give them a chance to explore their own emotions without judgment, and allow them to be excited for you in their own time.

25.

Overcome That Helpless Feeling

There will come a time in your pregnancy when you'll feel vulnerable to the powers that be, and you may find it to be a frightening experience. For example, you may order dinner from a restaurant and ingest a type of food poisoning. How can you protect your baby against the poison in your system? Perhaps you climb into a taxi or a bus, only to learn that the driver is completely reckless. If something happens to you, it happens to your baby.

You may develop a sense that you can't protect your unborn child. It's unsettling, it's terrifying, and it's magnified by your nature to want to nurture. Up until now, your only real physical concern was for yourself. In other words, every time you drank a cup of coffee, you may have thought about a recent report you read on the effects of caffeine, but you were probably not terribly concerned about it. Oh, how things have changed.

Both the inside and outside influences on your body become magnified when you are pregnant. Remember, however, that you were strong enough to have made it this far, and your body was strong enough to get pregnant. It is now strong enough to protect your baby.

In fact, in some ways, your body is stronger now than ever before—specifically to protect your baby. While you are busy worrying about what your body may or may not endure, your body has been busy getting ready to endure most anything that you get yourself into.

You have a baby to protect. Worrying won't help. Confidence in your own body's abilities and faith in the powers that be will see you through your pregnancy.

26.

A Politically Correct Pregnancy?

They're the flower children of the new millennium. They've not touched a sip of caffeine (including chocolate) since they were of childbearing age. They eat only raw, unprocessed, organic, vegetarian fare. They exercise three times a week and would never, ever, ever consider having fast food for dinner when they're pregnant.

It doesn't end there. They've hired a midwife for a natural home delivery and bought a swimming pool where they plan to give birth. No painkillers. No doctors. They'll bury the umbilical cord in the garden. The local cable channel will film the event.

They're wonderful. We applaud them. However, most of us are human. Carob just isn't the same as chocolate.

First of all, there is no such thing as the "perfect pregnant woman." Sure, there are those who run around in flowing dresses and hum Beethoven to their unborn children—but every pregnant lady has her secrets. Beethoven's music, it is rumored, is best enjoyed with a candy bar.

Secondly, "politically correct" changes from day to day and person to person. Remember that our own mothers were told not to gain more than ten pounds during their pregnancy. If you only gained ten pounds, everyone around you, including your mother and your doctor, would be concerned.

The most important thing is that you do what makes you feel comfortable. Forget the ever-changing rules and mores. You are your baby's mother. You only want what is best for his or her health. Unless you're spending your nights out drinking and carousing, you are taking care of your child the best way you know how to do.

That occasional cup of coffee won't kill you. Chocolate (in moderation) is a pregnancy "must." Beethoven isn't the only music you can hum to your unborn child. The decision to use painkillers during delivery is your own personal choice. Allow yourself some latitude during the nine long months of your pregnancy, and you will enjoy the experience much more than if you try to follow the "politically correct" image of what society wants you to be.

27.

Research "High-Risk" Pregnancy

If you're over the age of thirty-five, you are considered to be "high-risk." Never mind that you may be healthier than you were in your twenties. If you have ever lost a pregnancy, you may also now be high-risk. That doesn't count the millions of women who miscarry every year before they even know they are pregnant. If you are having twins, you are a high-risk pregnancy.

If you are considered to be a high-risk pregnancy, you need to listen very closely to your doctor's every word, but first ask your doctor exactly what high-risk means. If you are healthy, the word can be used loosely simply due to circumstance.

Do not allow this scare you. It is simply a way for the medical community to define their patients. You can, in fact, use the high-risk label to your advantage. Most likely, your insurance company will pay for extra ultrasounds, tests, and services due to your special circumstances. This will help to put your mind at ease through the course of your pregnancy.

28.

Use Your Wisdom to Your Advantage

Any woman over the age of thirty-five is considered to be an older mother and a high-risk pregnancy. Phooey!

Yes, there are certain risks involved. No, your body isn't quite as strong as it was ten years ago. Yes, it's important to undergo additional tests and listen very closely to your doctors.

However, look at the bright side. Many women over thirty-five years old are much more careful about how they act during their pregnancies than they would have been in their twenties. By their thirties, women are generally more nutrition-minded. They recognize consequences. They're a little more careful about physical exertion. On the other hand, they also understand the importance of regular exercise—especially when they're pregnant. Additionally, many women have come to grips with their own mortality. They've given up the notion that they need to go out and party every weekend.

One of the nicest advantages to slowing down physically is that it allows us to enjoy the moment more often. An "older" mother-to-be may savor (and remember) the special experience more than she would have in her twenties.

A woman over the age of thirty is also more likely to be established in a career when she becomes pregnant. This may mean that she faces a higher stress level from which she needs to protect herself. It should also mean that she has the resources to do so. A professional mother-to-be has already proven herself at the office. It's time to call in some favors, and then appreciate the fact that you have something to ponder other than your pregnancy aches and pains.

That is the key. You're a little wiser than you used to be. You know the value of regular exercise, eating well, and taking care of yourself. You have already proven yourself. It gives you an edge.

If you listen to your own wisdom, you may just be at a lower risk than you would have been if you were pregnant in your twenties. Just don't tell the doctor that—otherwise, you may not get those extra ultrasounds and tests that you're entitled to by virtue of age.

29.

Cause for Alarm?

Nearly fifty percent of all women bleed at some time during their pregnancy. This isn't necessarily cause for alarm.

In the very beginning of your pregnancy, you may notice spotting, or very light bleeding. This usually occurs around eleven to twelve days after fertilization. In fact, it may be around the same time that you are expecting your period. It's called "implantation bleeding," because it is a result of the fertilized egg burrowing into the uterine wall.

After the implantation bleeding, there may possibly be more. One minute you'll be happily pregnant, skipping around the house, deciding where to put the crib. Then you go to the bathroom, and suddenly it looks as though you have your period.

Yes, it can be a terrifying sight. Call your doctor or midwife immediately. Bleeding could be a sign of a miscarriage, ectopic (tubal) pregnancy, or another serious situation, especially if it is accompanied by severe abdominal pains or cramps. Do not, however, panic.

Bleeding does not necessarily mean that your pregnancy has come to an end.

Sometimes the bleeding is a result of a vaginal infection, a recent pap smear, or even sexual intercourse. Other times, no reason is discovered for the bleeding. Yet half of the women who bleed during the course of their pregnancies continue on to give birth to perfectly healthy babies.

Late in pregnancy, you may experience a discharge that is tainted with blood. This is actually called a "bloody show," and it is a sign that your mucus plug (which covers the opening of the cervix) has dislodged, and your cervix is beginning to soften or dilate in preparation for labor. The mucus plug may pass several weeks before your due date.

Again, if you do experience vaginal bleeding, always call your health care professional. Your doctor may want to run a couple of tests or suggest bed rest for a few days as a precaution. Take your doctor's advice. The odds are in your favor, and so is time.

Bleeding is not a sign of impending doom. It may simply be your body's way of telling you to slow down and take it easy while you're pregnant.

30.

Surviving a Miscarriage

Sadly enough, miscarriages do happen. To ease your mind, they only happen in fifteen percent of known pregnancies, so the odds are in your favor.

Although medical science cannot usually pinpoint any one reason for most miscarriages, it does indicate that chromosomal abnormalities may be a factor in over half of the cases. What does this mean?

If you have a miscarriage, you have most likely done nothing wrong. This is not your fault. Nor is it anyone else's fault.

Chromosomes are funny things. If they don't add up correctly, they may cause the fetus to be expelled. Many times (in at least fifty percent of all miscarriages), the woman's body terminates the pregnancy before she is even aware that she is pregnant.

Once you know that you are carrying a child, however, and have built up your hopes and dreams, a miscarriage takes on a whole new meaning. Unfortunately, there is nothing that can be said here to make you feel better. You need to mourn your loss in your own way, in your own time. Do not let anyone rush you. Do not feel obligated to "forget about it" and move on until you are ready.

Do understand that your partner and your friends love you—but they may not be certain how to help you. If they seem distant, it's only because they want to give you time to grieve. If they seem insensitive, they are probably scared to bring up the subject, because they don't want to hurt you even more. If they continuously talk about it, they are simply trying to make you feel better by letting you know how much they care about your loss.

Accept that people handle grief in different ways—and that includes you. Deal with your own emotions however you need to, without pressure or interference from well-meaning friends. Know that you did nothing wrong. You did nothing to deserve this. You will move past it to a perfectly healthy pregnancy—someday—when you're ready.

31.

Indulge Those Cravings

Donuts with pickles or hot dogs with salad dressing—at any time other than pregnancy, this would sound disgusting. For the pregnant woman, however, it can be "just what the doctor ordered"!

When you're pregnant, the cravings seem to blindside you and demand your attention immediately. Whoever expected that your body would be demanding Peking duck at two o'clock on a Tuesday morning?

Food cravings can be fun. When was the last time you were this whimsical with your appetite? You may not have even thought about peanut butter since you left home to go to college. Suddenly, you can't live another night without a peanut butter and banana sandwich. This can be the time of your pregnancy when you value your mate the most. Who else would drive to the local convenience store to buy you cookies after midnight?

You do know that nutrition counts. If a persistent craving for chocolate plagues you, it's time to see if fruit will satisfy your appetite instead. However, an occasional romp down the treat aisle can be good for the soul. Why not indulge your taste buds for a while?

On the opposite end of the spectrum are food aversions. Last week you may have eaten chicken salad three times for lunch. This week, the mere sight of chicken—or a salad—may make you queasy.

Don't push yourself to eat foods that spin your stomach around, no matter how healthy they may be. If greens send you running to the bathroom or milk makes your mouth pucker, then talk to your doctor. A vitamin supplement during the first couple of months can help balance your nutrition (at least until mid-pregnancy, when you will happily gobble down everything in sight).

Don't berate yourself for eating three donuts in a single sitting. It's done. You won't do it every day. Tomorrow you can pay more attention to what you eat. The point is to accept your cravings and yourself. You're working hard—you deserve a treat once in a while.

32.

Make the Most of Sleepless Nights

Counting sheep may become your favorite pastime during your pregnancy. In fact, one of the chief complaints among most mothers-to-be is that they simply cannot get a good night's sleep.

Early in the pregnancy, an expectant mother's own dreams, bladder, or hunger may wake her up time and time again. Once the pregnancy enters its third trimester and the baby is much larger, his or her kicking and positioning can become an issue. Add in leg cramps, heartburn, and hemorrhoids, and how is anyone expected to get any rest?

What may even be worse is that while you are chasing down the dream of a full night's sleep, your friends are laughing at the situation. "Wait until you have the baby," they say. "You'll never sleep again."

However, there are ways to help you capture that elusive slumber. Stay in a routine. Get up and go to bed at regular hours. Cut down on fluids in the evening. Stay away from caffeine past late noon. Exercise regularly. Late evening exercise should be light to avoid raising your heart rate before bedtime.

Keep your bedroom cool. Most people sleep best in temperatures below seventy degrees. Sleep on your left side. It takes the stress off the baby, your bladder, and important blood vessels that run down the back of your abdomen. Pillows are a girl's best friend. Tuck one under your head, as well as one between your legs to support your hip, one behind your back, or one under your growing belly.

If you find that you still can't sleep at night, why not take advantage of the extra time? Catch up on your reading, letter writing, or making notes in a journal. Rent that old movie you've always wanted to watch. (You don't need to watch the whole thing in one night.) Try getting a couple of chores done so that tomorrow you can take a catnap when the urge strikes. Using time now to give yourself time later is always satisfying.

33.
Don't Stress the Stress

Nearly a quarter of all mothers-to-be report some type of depressing feelings during their pregnancy. That's not surprising. While you're with child, you are dealing with hormonal influences the size of Mount Everest and—more importantly—lifestyle changes that dwarf the mighty mount. Of course you'll be a little weepy some days, and even sadder on other days. That is perfectly natural.

An unfortunate few expectant mothers, however, become consumed with these feelings of fear and hopelessness. They may experience anxiety attacks, compulsive disorders, or even clinical depression. There is something about the hormonal influences of pregnancy that can trigger a range of psychiatric disorders.

Lately, a lot of research has gone into depression during pregnancy. Recent studies have suggested that gestational depression (which peaks around the thirty-second week of pregnancy) is more common than its highly publicized cousin, postpartum depression.

The women at greatest risk for gestational depression are those who are predisposed to psychiatric disorders through heredity or their own personal history. However, not everyone has fair warning on this one, so you may want to keep tabs on your mental state. If you experience the following for more than two weeks, call your doctor.

- Persistent sadness or unhappiness
- Lethargy
- Loss of interest in previously enjoyed activities
- Sudden change of appetite or normal sleep patterns
- Difficulty concentrating

Chances are that your pregnancy will result in a couple of sad days—but those should be balanced by happy days. If you just can't shake the blues, or have had thoughts about harming yourself, it is important that you contact your doctor immediately. You are not the only one to experience gestational depression. Your doctor can help you.

34.

Help Your Other Children Adjust

Two-year-old Johnny realizes that he will no longer be the sole focus of your life. Seven-year-old Meghan and nine-year-old Zachary sense that they are "losing" their mother to a new baby. Fourteen-year-old Katie is confused by the fact that she's physically ready to become a mom herself, and now she'll soon have a baby brother.

Helping your other children adapt to a growing family can make them feel special. It can also take the pressure off you when the time comes to debut the newest addition.

Exactly how you approach your older child with the news depends on the child. A twelve-year-old daughter, for example, may be thrilled to hear about the development of the pregnancy every step of the way. Her three-year-old brother, on the other hand, is not likely to pay attention to the subtleties of a pregnancy, and nine months will feel like nine years to the toddler. It might be best to wait until you are in your third trimester to tell him the news.

Younger children may also still consider themselves to be the babies of the family. It's important that they understand that they will still have Mommy and Daddy to take care of them. Children can benefit from spending some time alone with each parent every day to reinforce their bonds.

If a toddler needs to be moved from the crib to make way for the new baby, start this process months before the delivery so that the older child views the move as an achievement. Otherwise, he or she may feel displaced from a security space—the crib—by the baby.

All children will bond better with baby if they are involved in the pregnancy. Allowing your kids to attend the ultrasound tests, hear the heartbeat, and witness the birth (or at least be present in the next room) are all things that can help children feel a connection with their soon-to-be sibling. At the same time, encourage your kids to develop and pursue their own interests. Let them know that their place in the family is safe and that they will always be loved.

Other ways to ease the transition include encouraging your older children to help make decisions for the new baby. Maybe they can narrow down baby's new name or help decorate the nursery. This is especially important if a sibling is going to share a room. The older sibling should have a say in the decor.

Get your older children involved in the pregnancy, allow them to help make decisions regarding their changing family, and encourage each child to be an individual. In this way, you will help your family to make a smooth transition to the days ahead.

35.

Mommy's Helpers

How will you handle another child on top of the ones you have? The first step is to involve them in the pregnancy. The next step is to make them proud of their new family role—turn them into Mommy's little helpers.

Talk to them about the importance of being older siblings. Check out books and videos on the subject from the library. Have a little party to celebrate their new role in the family.

Next, let them help you make decisions. They will feel more instrumental in their role as older brother or sister if they have helped to choose the layette. Start to train them in the basics of taking care of a baby. Dressing up a favorite doll can be a good way for a child to build anticipation for a new baby in the home. Children of any age can hand you a diaper or make funny faces at baby while he or she is in the bouncer and you are getting dressed in the same room.

Build excitement for a child's new role in the family. This will ensure that you get the help you need when the time comes.

36.

Enjoy Pregnancy Perks

Pregnancy privileges abound. Your local grocery store probably has a "baby club" promotional membership. It will include free stuff, coupons, free stuff, newsletters, and free stuff.

Your favorite pharmacy may provide designated parking spaces for expectant mothers. If not, they likely distribute "growing family" coupons for film development, vitamins, and moisturizers. Your obstetrician will always hand you a bag full of goodies that includes all sorts of offers for free pregnancy magazines and sample items.

Whether the perks of pregnancy mean that your husband washes the dishes at night or hundreds of dollars in discounts for you, enjoy them while they last. Don't forget about the little day-to-day perks. Buying a new wardrobe absolutely guilt-free has its joy. Having your husband and coworkers jump to your aid when you carry anything heavier than your purse is certainly a good thing.

It gets even better once you begin to show a definite pregnancy. A typical day may start this way. You take a taxicab to your local bank. A perfect stranger hails a cab and then gives it to you. Another one holds the elevator door for you while you're still two blocks away. A nice man insists that you step in front of him in the bank line. A sympathetic bank teller deletes the charges for two recently bounced checks because she remembers what it was like to be pregnant.

It's not a bad morning. In fact, it's not such a bad nine months. It is chock full of perks, and they are delightful, if you remember to relax and enjoy them.

37.

Avoid "Mommy-to-Be" Guilt

Television commercials, magazine advertisements, and books about pregnancy often paint a glorious picture of the blessed nine-month event. Isn't it true that all moms-to-be spend every single minute of all 280 days of gestation frolicking through the daisies with a glass of orange juice in one hand and a harpsichord in the other?

While it is certainly important to slow down your lifestyle to give yourself the opportunity to enjoy your pregnancy, nobody is expecting anybody to do anything for twenty-four hours a day. That's not to mention the fact that you still need to survive day-to-day life for each of those nine months—and life isn't always predictable.

That means that sometimes your lunch will be rushed and not as nutritious as you would like it to be. That unpaid bill will still weigh heavily on your mind. Your boss will have the same unreasonable demands that he always had. You may even need to miss a Lamaze class to attend your niece's soccer match. It's simply called "life."

Don't worry about not feeling guilty. You'll have plenty of time to feel guilty after the baby is born. You'll be a mother, which will be your job. You'll wonder, Is he crying too much at night or too little? Should he be crying at all? Why did I dress her in such a warm outfit on a summer day? He's crawling around on the floor, and I didn't mop today. She's spitting up again—was it something she ate? Oh no, what was it?

In the end, you'll come to the conclusion that you're human and you're doing the best you can. Why not adopt that attitude early on in your pregnancy, and spare yourself all of that mommy-to-be guilt?

38.

Appreciate All That "Good Advice"

There are days when you'll be running to your telephone to speed-dial some advice from Mom or Sis. You will thank heaven when they answer your call to tell you, "Yes, some women do lose hair during their pregnancy, and no, it doesn't mean that you have a strange prenatal scalp disease."

Girlfriends are among the best advisors, and you'll find yourself quizzing them on everything from pregnancy pimples to bladder control. Of course, your doctor should always be available to give you counsel. Do not be timid about calling him or her if you have a question. That is the doctor's job, and he or she should be happy to help. Most physicians would rather have a healthy patient with peace of mind than miss a symptom that may be a problem.

Then there is all that other "good advice." Upon seeing a pregnant woman, every other woman who has ever had a baby is suddenly an expert on gestation. Even more amazing are the number of male experts running around out there. You'll be swimming in a sea of pregnancy doctorates. Everyone from your waiter to your masseuse to the stranger at the theater will want to impart his or her knowledge.

What is a woman to do? Listen. Smile sweetly. Store away the gems of advice that you'll actually use—and ignore the rest.

Even if you're not receptive to unsolicited advice at the moment, it may come in handy later on. For instance, in month five, you may feel like a beached whale in your new swimsuit. The last thing you need is for some skinny woman to start talking to you (and thereby stand next to you and make you even look bigger). Who cares that Ms. Bag of Bones staved off stretch marks with cocoa butter cream? Yet a couple months later, when your belly starts to itch, and you're looking at the toll that this baby is taking on your own body, you may remember that the skinny woman was around forty and had twin toddlers. The cocoa butter advice can take on a whole new meaning.

Obviously, not every bit of information is a gem. The stranger who approaches you on the subway to tell you that your cup of tea, even if it's decaffeinated, can cause stunted growth in babies may have overheard that tidbit from his mother's uncle's stockbroker. Neither is all advice one-size-fits-all. Just because peppermint candies worked wonders on one woman's morning sickness doesn't mean that they will work for everyone—but why not try them if nausea is a big problem at the moment?

Can't hurt. Might help. Might not. Sift through the advice. Then call your mom, and see what she thinks.

39.

Belly Patting and Other Pregnancy Sports

In the convenience store, at the dry cleaner, and even in the waiting room of your dentist's office, people will want to touch your swollen belly. Some may come right up and put their hands on your abdomen. A few will ask your permission. Most will quietly assume that you'll say no, so they won't approach you, but they'll all be staring—and they'll all want to feel your little baby kick their palm from the womb.

Similarly, you will be surprised at the number of questions you receive from people you barely know. Why does your insurance agent care if you've bought larger shoes yet? Who is this new neighbor who wants to know if you've already chosen a preschool?

If you're the type of person who doesn't mind personal questions and people touching fairly intimate parts of your body, enjoy the attention. It can be a great experience to share with the world. In fact, that is why so many people are approaching you—they want to be involved, in some tiny way, in the miracle of pregnancy. Perhaps they are remembering their own pregnancies, when their babies were safe inside the womb. Maybe they are anticipating the time when they will have their own children.

Understand that others just want to share in your joy. However, do not feel obligated to offer your belly to every stranger who asks or to answer every question thrown your way. Pregnant women are already sharing their bodies with another human. They share their hopes and dreams with their partners. They share their experiences with their friends. They tell their concerns to their doctors. No mother-to-be is obligated to placate the masses or to tolerate intrusive behavior. If you're not comfortable with all of the poking and prodding, simply turn away. Although it may be well intended, no one has the right to touch you without permission.

You have every right not to participate if you don't want to. After all, how do you think someone else would react if you quizzed her on her shoe size or groped his stomach in the grocery store?

40.

Enjoy a New Bond with Your Parents

Mothers relate to other mothers, and they relate nearly as well to mothers-to-be. As your pregnancy progresses, you will slowly be accepted by the other moms in the world. You'll gain insight into the lives of your parent friends. This not only gives you a lot more to talk about, but it adds a new dimension to your friendships.

The most important friendship that you'll strike up through your pregnancy will be the one with your own parents. Whether you are already best friends with your own mother or you moved halfway across the country to get away from her, she may be the first person you want to call when you have a question. She will be thrilled that, after all these years, you are asking for her advice. After all, who is better qualified to mentor you through this unpredictable pregnancy stuff than your mother?

Nearly as dedicated to your cause as your family will be the father-to-be's family. A renewed relationship will probably also extend to your in-laws.

Your own parents and in-laws have been waiting a very long time for this day. All parents want a grandchild, regardless of whether it is their first or their thirty-first. They may also have been anticipating the time when you and your partner fully understand all that they did for you when you were kids. Most of all, they want to share the special bond of parenthood with you. There are so many tips to give and secrets to share.

Pregnancy is a great vehicle for striking up a friendship. That is especially true if the friendship that you make is one with your own parents.

41.
Why Isn't He Excited?

You spend your days examining the nutritional value of every morsel of food that crosses your lips. You're investigating Lamaze classes, buying baby name books, and trying to figure out a color scheme for the nursery. However, aside from last week, when he wouldn't let you carry the groceries into the house (which was sweet), he's barely mentioned the life growing inside of you. It seems as though he doesn't even realize that he's going to be a father in a few months.

If this is his first child, the chances are that he doesn't, really, realize that he's going to be a father in a few months. Pregnancy, of course, makes a much greater impact on mothers. Fatigue, nausea, and their ever-changing bodies remind them of their condition several times a minute. First-time mothers are especially preoccupied with unanswered questions about how their bodies are going to respond to pregnancy.

Your mate, on the other hand, can quite easily forget about the whole thing for long stretches at a time. He's not besieged with physical reminders. His life is pretty much the same as it always has been. Additionally, your man may need time to let the news sink in. He's heard a hundred times that his life is about to change and will never be the same. What if he likes his life as it is?

He's also heard the same horror stories that you have. His buddy's girlfriend had a horrendous labor period. His boss's wife was prescribed bed rest for six months. His mechanic's partner just had triplets last week! So while he may not be thinking about the baby twenty-four hours a day, seven days a week, as you are, he probably is slowly beginning to absorb his upcoming role of fatherhood—and there's a lot of information to wade through.

He may not be excited yet, but he will be. The baby may not even become a reality for him until the day he holds his own child in his arms. On that day, he will be absolutely ecstatic.

42.

Adjusting Emotionally Together

One evening, you're feeling fragile. You just want to nest. You're envisioning a quiet night of old movies while snuggled up on the sofa with your lover. When you arrive home from work, he's on the phone arranging to meet his buddies for martinis to celebrate the pregnancy.

The following morning, you feel like Superwoman, ready to conquer the world. Your man is now trailing your every move, concerned that you're taking on too much. Later in the afternoon, you want to go out and buy baby clothes, but he just wants to sit home and watch the game.

It may be that you both simply need time to adjust to your impending lifestyle, and you may need to do it in different ways. While you can't wait to go out together and buy baby clothes, all he can think about is the fact that he'll actually have to dress someone other than himself in the morning—and dressing himself may already be a huge responsibility in his book. Don't even mention that some outfits come with snaps for easy diaper changes.

There's also the chance that he is not exactly sure how to read your emotions. You probably are a bit moody these days. He may feel that saying nothing or avoiding you is the best tack to take. For instance, when you told him that you outgrew your favorite "fat clothes," did he really try to console you with a carton of ice cream? He sure did.

Soon, your emotional lows and highs will (most likely) find a middle ground together. At the very least, you'll learn to respect each other's responses—and maybe even laugh at yourselves in the process.

43.

Bonding with Baby

On one of those typically wistful days during your pregnancy, you may envision that single magical moment when you first lay eyes on your little angel. You will finally meet the person with whom you've been sharing the most intimate of homes for nine months. Your caregiver will lay your darling gently on your shoulder. You'll feel a soft breath and take one look at that heavenly face. Suddenly, you will swell with a sense of love so complete that you are enlightened to the meaning of love for the very first time.

After all, don't all new mothers fall in love with their babies instantly? Many do—and they say that it's a sweet experience. Many fathers are also transformed by that shining moment. However, not everyone experiences the earth-shattering feeling of unconditional love with one look at a pink, wrinkly face. You may not reach nirvana the first time you look at your child. You may not even reach it the second time, the third, or afterward. That is perfectly okay, and it is more common than you may think.

The word "bonding" does not refer to a single moment. It does not even necessarily refer to your emotions. It simply means the way mothers and their newborns learn to synchronize their behaviors to each other. The key word is "learn." Learning takes time. The relationship will develop as a continuing process. Bonding does not happen instantly.

Some women grow to love their children as they get to know them. Their love is just as strong as those who fall in love with their babies at first sight. A growing love does not mean that your bond with your child is any less significant than if you had fallen in love immediately.

Remember that your body will be in a hormonal, physical, and emotional spin for a few months yet. Even if this is not your first child, your world will change in every possible way. Many parents are nervous and exhausted during the initial stages of a new baby's life. It's no wonder that some new mothers and fathers need time to adjust before they can relax and actually enjoy their babies!

It may take a few weeks, or even months, before you truly grow to love your child as fully as you thought you might when you first saw him or her. Relax, and let it happen at its own pace. Once it does, you will truly learn to understand how precious that love can be.

44.

See the Humor of the Couvade Syndrome

You're the one lugging twenty-some extra pounds around every day. Why is it that he is so tired all the time? It seems that he matches you craving per craving—and he's nauseated nearly every morning. If an alien species were to observe our race, they might just determine that it's the human male who bears the offspring, since some men seem to have more symptoms than the women. This is known as Couvade syndrome, or "sympathetic pregnancy." The phrase is derived from the French root word *couver*, which means "to hatch."

It has been estimated that nearly eighty percent of fathers-to-be develop some pregnancy symptoms. The most common symptom is weight gain. For the record, nearly all men gain weight during their wives' pregnancies. Other symptoms can include nausea, indigestion, insomnia, toothaches, back pain, stomach spasms, and even moodiness. Some men even experience "labor pains."

No one knows for certain what causes Couvade syndrome. It tends to begin around month three of a pregnancy and continues until birth. On one hand, it's nice to have somebody so empathetic to your discomfort that they're quite literally feeling it as their own pain. On the other hand, you know that you are really the one going through this, so why do you have to listen to his complaints?

Try to remember that your mate truly is in discomfort. Whether his aches are psychosomatic (as some doctors maintain) or physical, he really does feel your pain. Then remind him that it is your pain.

You're the one who still deserves the foot rubs and the long, warm baths. Give him extra attention and reassurance when he doesn't feel well, but don't let his newfound pimples and mood swings convince you that he is the one who needs to be taken care of right now.

45.

Accept Some Jealousy with the Territory

Pregnant women steal the spotlight. They don't mean to. It's just that everyone else in the room—including all of those women who have been pregnant—is wondering how it is that you manage to look so radiant while you're just a little busy creating another human being inside of you.

Even if you can't see your own amazing beauty at the moment and all of the attention that it brings, others do see it. Sometimes this may evoke a little envy in those around you. Your girlfriends may long for their pregnant days (whether those days are in the distant past or the future). They may wish that they, too, were enjoying this special time of their life. Anyone standing by your side, in fact, may become invisible when you enter a room and everyone flocks to you to ensure your comfort and offer you food.

Your partner may feel a little forgotten. He can barely go to work, the gym, or his favorite cocktail hour without every close associate asking, "So how is your lovely bride doing with her pregnancy?" His female friends may be especially interested in your progress. He just wants to discuss the latest baseball scores or his theory on the current presidential election, and people will listen politely for a moment and then interrupt with, "Do you know if it's a boy or girl?" "Is the mommy getting enough rest?" or "Are you sure that you should be here instead of at home with her?"

Remember that your friends and family may get a little jealous of you during this time. They deserve some extra time and attention—especially from the person who seems to be getting all of the attention these days.

46.

Build a Support System

There will be days when your pregnancy is all that you can think about, dream about, and worry about. Fortunately, almost all of the mothers you know will be happy to talk about the symptoms and side effects of being pregnant. You can call them with the slightest of complaints, and they'll gladly dole out advice and sympathy. These are the people who will comprise a large part of your future. While it may seem difficult to comprehend at this stage, your entire social circle will shift once you've had kids.

Yes, your childless friends will still be friends, and you will make it to the annual barbecue and the local holiday party. In fact, make it a point to spend some one-on-one time with these people so that those relationships do not wither. However, once you have had your beautiful baby, it's your parent friends who will become increasingly invaluable. The same woman who taught you how to massage your temples for headache relief when you were two months pregnant will be the same mom you call for a cure for colic when your baby is screaming in the middle of the night. She will then be the one you go to visit regularly, because she helps with your toddler.

Of course, your family will make up a large part of your support group. Your own mother and your partner's mother, and both your sisters and brothers, will all start to play a more significant role in your life. They will be the ones to stop by and actually help to carry your baby around when your arms have become numb.

Do try to be careful of whom, exactly, you lean on during your pregnancy. Unfortunately, some people (and they may even be your close friends or family members) are negative by nature. If you call them because you are concerned about aches and pains, they'll immediately have you believing that they are anything but minor.

Your friends are going to shift at this time of your life. Why not make it a change for the positive and build yourself a strong support system for the future?

47.

Give Yourself Permission to Dream

Sometimes we're scared to let our imaginations run and play. For instance, you may want to fantasize about dressing up your darling red-headed daughter in a pink ballerina tutu for Halloween—but…what if "she" turns out to be a blond-haired little boy?

Don't restrict yourself from dreaming. It is one of the most delightful qualities of being a human. Instead, why not permit yourself to dream freely and have many different dreams at once?

You may see a magazine ad for a wispy-haired little girl with big blue eyes and pink cheeks. Is she the spitting image of your darling daughter-to-be—that girl who will grow into the tutu? The next page may feature a photo of a dark-skinned little boy with brown eyes and a smile to melt your heart. Is that what your future son will look like? Can you imagine him in a cowboy costume?

Who says that you can only have one fantasy baby? Who says that you can only have one baby? You're young. When your baby is finally born, you might actually recognize a combination of features from your many different visions along the way.

Similarly, you may find yourself wondering about temperament, personality, or talents. Again, let yourself fantasize while you are pregnant. Is she spunky? Is he cautious? When the baby comes out to meet the world, his or her personality will slowly unveil itself. She will no doubt surprise you in many ways. Then again, he may turn out to be that same little musician you've envisioned.

Perhaps your dreams are not so specific and you just want to feel the skin of your newborn snuggled against your breast. So why not go to sleep with that thought in your mind? Allow yourself to dream. The more dreams we have, the more alive we become, and one of the best parts of being alive is having dreams.

48.

Breaking the News to Your Boss

You may be blessed to work at a family-oriented business. There are a few enlightened companies that support committed, personal relationships, embrace children, and may even provide child-care services. Many other businesses may not be quite so enthusiastic about new-parent employees, but they often do value their staff and will support you during your pregnancy and maternity leave.

Hopefully, you are fortunate enough to have a family-friendly work environment. Many pregnant women, however, do not. Even if you believe that your company will support you, it is important that you understand your boss's position on maternity leave before you announce your condition.

This is not to suggest that you mislead your employer in any way. It is, however, a good idea to know your company's policy—as well as your own intentions—before you notify the workplace.

The moment you announce that you're pregnant, there will be one question on everyone's mind: "Is she coming back after the baby?"

Before you shrug that question off with "Of course I am," be certain of your own position. Talk to other moms, those who work both inside and outside of the home. Ask them their opinions. Weigh your own priorities.

There may actually be no decision. If your household is dependent upon your salary for survival, then you will work. If your work is hazardous, then you will quit tomorrow—and forget about waiting another day.

Of course, there are all sorts of places to meet in the middle. Can you telecommute? Job share? If you are planning to continue work, who will handle your duties when you're gone? Who will take care of your baby while you're earning a salary? You may even find that child care takes so much of your paycheck that you're better off staying home for a couple of years.

Telling your coworkers about your pregnancy may be a delicate situation. Make sure that you have the answers to the questions— both yours and theirs—before you make the announcement.

49.

Respect Stay-at-Home Moms

In the eighties, women were expected to "do it all." Women regularly bragged at the office that they started labor during a Monday morning business meeting, spent the next twelve hours clearing their desks, drove straight to the hospital, had a kid, and made it back to work for Tuesday's regular office happy hour.

In the nineties, women realized the value of those initial few hours with their babies. Those hours stretched into days, weeks, and years. Today, many moms are choosing to spend that time exclusively with their kids. They've heard the advice over and over again to enjoy each age, because it is fleeting. They want to be there to help shape their children during every stage of development.

Not everyone can do this. If your family would need to sell all their possessions and move to the nearest YMCA to survive on one salary, then staying at home is simply not an option. If you have always been driven by your career and would suffer for a long stretch of time without it, then being a stay-at-home mom is not for you.

Besides, you will have many other types of lessons to teach your child down the line. Studies show that youngsters who grow up with daycare are ultimately just as well adjusted as those with stay-at-home moms.

As a compromise, many women are opting to forego the family extras or take a job that offers flexibility to spend more time with their children. It's not necessarily that they believe they will deprive their children if they work a full-time job. Many of these women shift priorities because they do not want to deprive themselves. They've listened to the advice of the masses, and as the masses will tell you, enjoy these years, because they truly are fleeting.

50.

Play Give-and-Take at the Office

Your thoughts are focused on one thing these days, and your coworkers have probably noticed. Most of your office mates will be thrilled for you. They may understand about all of those sick days. They turn their heads the other way as you slide out of staff meetings to use the ladies' room (again and again). Very few would even think to object when you schedule your ultrasound exams during office hours.

Just be careful not to take advantage of their kindness and tolerance. Nine months takes a lot of patience on anyone's part (especially yours, of course). Even though you're pregnant, you are still being paid the same wage as before the pregnancy.

At the same time, take care not to over-commit yourself to too many responsibilities. If you find that you are wearing yourself thin in any one area of your life, whether it is your career or your pregnancy, make it a point to step back and reevaluate your priorities. You may come to realize that you need to cut back on your work duties or hours—or you may find the opposite. Perhaps you've been neglecting your career and cheating your employer.

Work at striking a balance between your job and your soon-to-be profession of motherhood. After all, you may well be depending on your coworkers while you're away on maternity leave, and they will certainly be depending on you to guide them through that time (and beyond, if you decide not to return to the office).

There is only so much you can do right now. Try not to over-commit yourself in any one important area, for everyone's sake.

51.

Take a Step Back

We're women. It's a biological fact that our brains work differently than men's brains. It is also a fact that because of this, we often experience emotion at a higher and deeper level than men. Occasionally, our emotions sway even more strongly than usual. Instead of just surprising our friends and partners with our passions, we may even surprise ourselves.

Up until now, many of your emotional explosions may have depended on the time of the month. Think back to how that little surge of hormones may have affected you in the past. Imagine what the flood of those same hormones might be doing to you now.

We often realize that we're overreacting on the spot. Yes, it does seem silly to toss the entire meatloaf into the garbage just because we added too much tomato sauce to the recipe—but you do it anyway. Someone has to teach that darned chunk of meat a lesson!

Other times, your emotions simply take control. The saga of your anger (fear, pain, jealousy) plays over and over—like the proverbial broken record—through your mind. You feel muddled. You can't think about anything else.

That is the time when you truly need to step back and take a deep breath. It's okay to replay the experience that is so bothersome to you, and it is even a good idea to talk about it with someone on the outside of the event. However, give yourself some time before you react.

Why not take three days? At the end of that time, you might just realize that your boss was only questioning your progress, not your work. It may become clear that your mother-in-law really does care about your health and was not judging your eating habits, or that your mate was actually complimenting your new outfit—not pointing out that it's a size 16.

By refusing to act on your initial rage, you're taking back control of your emotions. In this way, you'll make your pregnancy that much easier.

52.

Consider Yourself Truly Blessed

Yes, there may be millions of women every year who conceive a child—and you are one of them. There are also millions of women who wish that they could conceive a child. Many women are past their physical ability. Some have an unfortunate medical history that makes pregnancy impossible. Others have simply been trying and trying and trying.

Don't take your good fortune for granted. No, your body will never be exactly the same. Yes, your life is about to spin 180 degrees. Soon you will be the slave of a tiny, squirming blob of flesh. You will be awake all night, falling asleep all day, and wondering what your "normal life" was like. Then you'll sit down in your rocking chair and that darling will fall sound asleep against your chest. At that moment, you'll understand what your life is all about.

Until that day, try to remember that you are now experiencing the most magical part of womanhood. You are creating a little angel inside your own body. You are truly blessed.

53.

Relax During the Middle Months

Is she or isn't she? A lot of people may be staring at you from afar and wondering, "Is she carrying a child, or has she simply tossed back too many milkshakes since I've seen her last?" What may be even worse, in your mind, is that the people who don't know you also don't know that you're pregnant. They'll simply assume that you always look like this—sporting an extra twenty pounds around the middle.

So? This is temporary. More important, you're beautiful. How do you know that those same people you meet now won't see you again after your baby is born and think that you actually looked better when you were pregnant?

The second trimester may feel discouraging as you try to manage your growing waistline, but most women feel that this is the best time of a pregnancy. Month four brings an end to morning sickness, along with a new energy. Many women report that they feel healthier in their middle months of pregnancy than ever before. They have a renewed sense of self and peacefulness.

This is the time to take a vacation with your man. It will probably be the last time—for a very long time—that the two of you can sneak away alone together. Whether you want to conquer that dream trip that you have been discussing, or if you only escape for a weekend, take advantage of the middle months. Use this trimester to reconnect with your own emotions, with your partner, and with your common goals. Take slow moments to truly appreciate your pregnancy, and quietly start to prepare for the future of your newborn.

The nausea is gone. The major aches and pains are yet to come. Relax and enjoy this period of your pregnancy.

54.

Is It a Boy or a Girl?

It's the first question that everyone will ask you upon hearing the good news: Is it a boy or a girl? It may even be the first thought that crosses your mind once you learn that you're pregnant. Then again, it may be the very last thing you want to know.

In that respect, you control the situation. Although most first- and second-time parents can't wait to find out if they will be buying blue booties or pink ribbons, veteran child-bearers frequently revel in the suspense of the baby's sex. It adds a little more excitement to the moment. Besides, boy or girl, the most important consideration is your baby's health. At the time you give birth, the only things that you will really care about will be your child's first breath, followed by a finger and toe count. Do you really want to know your child's sex?

Okay, you do—and you want to know at the first possible opportunity. Perhaps you are desperately hoping for a specific gender. In that respect, you have no control of the situation. What you do have, however, is the innate ability to love your child unconditionally—male or female.

Some women learn this lesson over time. One woman urgently wanted to have a baby girl. She was raised in a family of sisters. What did she know about boys? When she had her son, she was amazed by what a doting father her husband became. She doubted that he would have been so involved if she had borne a daughter. Another mother had her heart set on a son. She wanted to play in the dirt and collect bugs. Her little girl was the spitting image of the mother. The two became constant companions and the best of friends. They read novels together, painted pictures of unicorns, and even played in the dirt.

If you've already knitted a blanket in one color or another, it may be a disappointment to learn that your baby is of the opposite sex. Disappointment is okay. It's even expected. Eventually, your disappointment will give way to exaltation.

Pardon the cliché, but sometimes what is meant to be is truly meant to be. The bottom line is that you will love your child deeply, regardless of his or her sex. In fact, you may even come to change your mind about what you thought you wanted.

55.

There's No Such Thing as a Perfect Parent

Suddenly, they're everywhere. Drive past a school at three in the afternoon, and they're there. Jog through a local park in the morning—there they are. The library, the grocery store, the bank—there are mommies doting on their children. "Perfect parents," you might think to yourself. The sight can be breathtaking—especially when you're pregnant.

There's the woman walking down the street. The chubby fingers of a little boy rest in her left hand. Her right hand squeezes the palm of a little girl. What about your neighbor, who spends most evenings on a porch swing, cradling her newborn in her arms? Both of these moms have wide grins, and seemingly all of the patience in the world. The sight can be intimidating—especially when you're pregnant.

What if you don't become that all-loving parent that you envision? Babies don't come with instruction manuals. When are you supposed to feed a baby and when do you put him down for a nap?

How will you know what to do if (when) your baby is screaming all night long and nothing seems to help? Who is going to teach her to talk? What if you just don't like this whole parenting business?

Take heart that every one of these "perfect parents" that you see had the exact same fears as you do. It is more than likely that not one of them considers herself to be a perfect parent. In fact, there is no such thing.

You will probably end up feeding your child fast food from time to time. At some point, you'll turn your back for a second, and your son will fall down. No matter how many discussions you have with your teenage daughter about smoking and drinking, she will probably try one or the other at some point.

However, even without a manual, you will be a splendid parent. You have two of the most valuable tools in your hands: mothering instinct—the strongest intuition that you'll ever have, which will tell you most of what you need to know when the time comes; and an undeniable love for the well-being of your child. Even if you are an imperfect parent, you will have a perfect love for your children—and that is all you need to be a "perfect parent."

56.

Will You Become Your Parents?

Carrying a child will open a floodgate of memories from your own childhood. Most of those visions will be sweet. All of them will have one thing in common—you'll look back on your younger years in an entirely different way. Instead of seeing things strictly through a child's eyes, you'll now see things through your child's eyes—and you'll wonder if you want your child to experience his or her growing days the same way that you did.

You may decide that long walks through the woods or visits to the zoo are some of your fondest recollections. Your child should definitely grow up with those. You may also remember that spankings were some of your worst experiences. "Okay," you decide. "No heavy-handed discipline."

At this time, you may start to become critical of the way that your own parents raised you. Fortunately, you will now also have a strong ability to put yourself in your folks' shoes. After all, in our parents' day, spankings were a sign of love. They regularly said, "This will hurt me more than it will hurt you," and they meant it. They were simply trying to teach us rules, like "Do not run into the street!" It was for our own safety.

Similarly, you may love the way that your mother brought you a glass of milk every night when she put you to bed. That's a lovely sentiment that you'd like to continue with your own children. You may also remember the night when she publicly humiliated you because you sneaked out of the house to meet your boyfriend at a party. "I hope that my daughter doesn't try the things that I tried," you'll muse. You will suddenly understand her hysteria at finding her fourteen-year-old out at a party at midnight.

So when you ask yourself: "Will I become my mother? Will he become his father?" often the answer is, "Yes. If you're lucky." The only difference is that with each generation, we gain a little more experience and a little more wisdom. The biggest similarity is that you will love your child with the same fierce abandon that your parents loved you. Because of that, you will do what is right for your child in the best way that you know how—just as your mother did.

57.

Consider Bed Rest as an Opportunity

Some view it as a jail sentence: bed rest—for three days, three weeks, three months, or more. It can be incredibly painful to lose one's freedom. Suddenly, all you can think about are the things that you would be doing if you were up and about. After procrastinating for a year, you really were going to re-grout the bathtub this weekend. Really, you were—and now you can't!

Nearly twenty percent of pregnant women are prescribed bed rest each year for various reasons, and there are different degrees of immobility. Many ladies may take a shower, make a sandwich, and sit up for limited periods of time. Others cannot. Some will need the professional care that a hospital has to offer.

If you have been grounded, here's a question: How many projects have you fantasized about completing "if only you had the time"? Forget the bathroom grout. What about all of those things that you can do while you're stationary?

This is a great opportunity to read all of those pregnancy books—and how many other books have you wanted to read? Why not take this time to learn Spanish, or finally study the market for exporting those designer handbags that you intend to create someday? What about organizing all your photographs in albums and scrapbooks?

Reading is one way to pass the time. Writing, watching classic movies, calling old friends, and sewing can be others. Still, aside from occasional bouts of boredom, you may encounter loneliness. Yesterday you were a social butterfly. Today you're not allowed to step outside your front door.

After a week, you will probably call every single friend and coworker with pleas to come visit you. Try organizing a "takeout dinner in bed" party for your girlfriends or a regular day each week for your friends to hang out at your place. Have your sweetie pick up some wine for them, juice for you, and snacks. Then he can check out. (He will be thrilled at the opportunity to spend some time with the guys and not worry about entertaining you for the evening.) The best part about being in bed is that nobody will expect you to clean your house.

While bed rest can be frustrating, it can also be an opportunity to grow, relax, and reflect. As Americans, we forget to slow down and enjoy what we have. Sometimes, we need a higher power to tell us to stop! Slow down! Enjoy the moment. After all, you'll never be here—at this precise time of your life—again.

58.

Embrace Embryo Gymnastics

If this is your first child, you will most likely not recognize that initial "flutter" as the baby's kicks. Quite frankly, it can feel just like indigestion. In fact, you're much more likely to blame that tickling sensation on the taco that you ate for lunch than your baby.

Then one day you will realize, perhaps with a giggle or a tear, that "Hey! That's my little one moving around inside of me!" With every ounce the fetus gains, the kicks become stronger. Soon, they become loving (if not startling) reminders of the fact that you are actually carrying another human being inside of your womb.

For many women, this is when the pregnancy becomes "real." Also for many women, this is the perfect time to start recording a journal of your baby's movements. This "kick diary" will accomplish two purposes. First, it will tell you the times when your child is most active. These will most likely be after you have eaten a meal and—for some reason—at night, when you are trying to sleep. That means that the diary will also reveal when the "safest" time is for you to rest without being interrupted from within. Soon, you'll be able to predict your child's rhythm. There will be certain hours when the baby is quite calm (often, when you are walking), and there will be other times when the baby is quite active.

A diary will also show you how those reassuring nudges can start to reveal your darling's personality. The baby may "dance" to certain types of music, kick your belly when you wear tight waistbands, or nap through certain TV shows.

Eventually, you may notice that your baby has hiccups. Do not let this alarm you. By all medical accounts, the hiccups are not painful to the baby. Consider them just another beautiful reminder of the magical life within you. Then jot down the time of the hiccups in your journal as more evidence that your baby is growing perfectly healthy.

59.

Multiple Birth, Multiple Joy

Your first words will be similar to "Oh, dear Lord!" upon hearing the news that you are having more than one baby. That exclamation will be followed by a pause while the reality of the situation sinks in. You may walk into a regularly scheduled doctor's appointment wondering what color booties to buy, and then walk out wondering how you'll ever be able to afford booties—or how you'll manage to get four (or more) booties on four (or more) sets of wiggling toes.

What toll will twins or triplets take on your body? Do you have enough strength to nurture multiple fetuses? (Yes, you do.) Will you ever be able to fit into your jeans again? (Maybe, maybe not—but you run the same risk with any pregnancy. The good news is that jeans are sold in various sizes.)

According to the parents of twins, two babies truly are harder to care for than one. That may not be a surprise to most of us. However, those very same parents report that two toddlers may actually be easier to care for than one—well, maybe not easier, but not as difficult as you might imagine. In a year or two, the kids can play together and don't expect you to be their constant companion. As they grow, they will most likely form a strong bond of friendship. Don't we all want a friend who truly understands us? Despite their closeness throughout the years, they will maintain their own distinct personalities.

It may take a while to get past the initial shock. In the end, however, when you look at those two (or more) adorable faces looking up at you, you will be absolutely delighted that you had more than one child.

60.

Naming Your Baby

It may be the easiest part of your pregnancy, or it may be the hardest. For many couples, naming their baby is a drawn-out decision. Baby naming can be quite a challenging sport.

She may want to name her daughter Casey, since she, herself, called her own doll-babies by that name when she was five years old. He hates the name. Why can't they name the baby after his dear mother, Gertrude?

Then comes the sense of duty. Quite often, people feel obligated to name their offspring after respected (and/or deceased) relatives. That seems to be when every family member has an opinion. Why should your son bear the name of his father's father? What's wrong with your father's name? You must love your father-in-law more than your own father. What kind of daughter are you?

Your child's name needs to be approved by only two people: you and the father. So what if your sister doesn't like the name? Who cares if there is already a Devon in the family? There will be a dozen

Devons at your kid's school. Why name your child after your grandparent, if you don't actually like the name itself?

Remember that the name of your child is the decision of you and your partner. If the two of you vehemently disagree, give it some time. A name that one of you refuses to budge on may not seem like such a great name a couple of weeks down the line. Use the power of middle names to your advantage, and remember that you only need to please yourselves, not your child. After all, no matter what you name your children, they are sure to turn to you in perhaps eleven years and tell you that they hate their names anyway.

61.

Appreciate Tests and More Tests

As your pregnancy progresses, so will the frequency of visits to the obstetrician's office. Near the end, you will find yourself finishing lengthy magazine articles in the waiting room that you actually started a couple of visits beforehand. You're there for tests, tests, and more tests. It can be frustrating, but you should be thankful for every frustrating moment of those tests. They have saved the lives of many, many babies, and even the lives of some mothers.

Each of your office visits will consist of urine tests (to check for protein to make sure that you are not developing toxemia), a jump on the scale, and a blood pressure reading. A vaginal examination may or may not be a part of your normal office procedure, although an initial culture (similar to a pap smear) will be taken to ensure an absence of cervical cancer and STDs.

On one of your first visits, your blood will be run to check for things such as hormone levels and HIV. Depending on your situation, you may also receive a host of other blood tests. The first is a chorionic villi sampling (CVS) that checks for genetic abnormalities. There is also the alpha-fetoprotein test (often called the "triple test") that shows whether the spinal column and brain are developing normally. For the glucose tolerance test, to make sure that you have not developed gestational diabetes you must first drink a pint of chalky liquid.

Due to your age, circumstance, or the result of a prior test, you may be prescribed an amniocentesis. Yes, that's the long needle. No, it doesn't hurt nearly as much as you imagine. Some women barely feel it. The procedure (used to detect Down syndrome and other genetic abnormalities) is nothing compared to the two-week wait to get the results.

Results are the sticky part. More than one woman has had a negative prognosis and still had a perfect healthy baby. If your doctor tells you that he or she wants to run more tests—and not to worry in the meantime—try to follow that advice and relax a little. A suspicious test result does not necessarily mean a negative outcome.

Ultrasounds (or sonograms) will be your favorite tests—except for all of the water that you need to drink prior to the test. This is where you will come face to face (or leg or buttocks) with your little angel. It may also be the first time that your partner realizes, "Hey! There's a child growing inside of you." Thanks to all of those tests, you're both going to be just fine.

62.

Get Comfortable, Girl!

Shoes, rings, waistbands—sometimes they can hurt a pregnant woman's swollen and sensitive body. Why not get rid of them all?

When you consider that your blood volume may increase as much as forty percent, which means that your circulatory system is both working harder and slowing down, it makes sense that your body will be swollen. There are a few things that you can do every day to help alleviate the swelling. They are walking, resting, and drinking water.

Try to walk fifteen to twenty minutes a day in a cool area. This helps to relieve some of the swelling, because as the leg muscles move, the blood is forced back up toward the heart.

Also, rest with your legs elevated when you can. Sleep on your side to decrease the amount of weight placed on major arteries.

Drink at least eight to ten glasses of water (or juice or milk) a day. Although it sounds counterproductive, drinking more fluids will actually help to flush out your system and alleviate swelling.

The first thing that any pregnant woman needs to do is to find herself several pairs of wide, comfortable, low-heeled shoes. In fact, forget about high heels for a while. They will hurt your feet and your back by throwing your spine even further out of alignment. You don't need them while your body is growing. (By the way, keep in mind that you will need to buy a larger pair of wide, comfortable, low-heeled shoes in your last trimester.)

Secondly, avoid anything that is tight or irritating. The exception may be pregnancy pantyhose or a "belly brace," which can be comfortable once one gets used to it. Pull off those rings, waistbands, and belts. You don't need them.

However, don't be tempted to slough off your seatbelt. You need it. The highest cause of death to pregnant women is automobile accidents. Even if you were to survive an accident, you would never forgive yourself if a seatbelt could have made a difference to the health of your baby. No matter how much your belly may protest, do protect it with a seatbelt.

There are some things that a woman should forego during pregnancy. There are other things that she should not.

63.

Free Your Own Inner Child

During our journey into adulthood, we have learned to control our emotions. Without this suppression mechanism, one might, for example, give way to a temper tantrum upon receiving a speeding ticket. Others might be tempted to call in sick to go rolling around in the grass on every warm spring day.

As adults, we also forget to marvel at butterflies and truly appreciate the softness of a down comforter. The smell of home-baked bread reminds us to eat lunch. What about savoring the aroma for the scent itself?

That is one of the most beautiful things about pregnancy. Your emotions are on high alert, and your senses are changing on a continuous basis. Allow yourself to relish these moments. Watch the butterfly for as long as you can see it. Inhale the sweet smell of that fresh bread. Take this opportunity to enjoy the experiences of life that we so often take for granted. It really is not such a sin to roll around in the grass on a beautiful spring day—even if you have to play hooky every now and then to do so.

64.

Ask for What You Need

You are having a baby. People will buy you gifts. Why not help them out by allowing a friend to host a baby shower? This is not the time to be bashful. On the contrary, you will be doing your friends a favor by letting them know what you need—and by the way, you're going to need lots of stuff.

Although most babies can live to be a ripe old age without ever once sitting in a bouncer, your best friend will swear that it is the single item that saved her sanity. Ditto for your sister's swing and your aunt's butterfly mobile that plays music for ten straight minutes.

First, ask for what your baby needs. Then ask for what you want. If something looks like it might make your life a little bit easier, put it on your registry. Don't be shy. Your friends and family would much rather get you something that they know you want and will use than risk being the fourth person to give you a bassinet.

The question here may be: how do you know what will make your angel happy? Will the baby prefer an activity station or a playpen? What will be used and what will just take space? The answer is that you just won't know until the child arrives and tells you. Each baby is an individual. A toy that occupies one gleefully may scare another.

This is another time that you will be grateful to all of your mommy friends who pass around their used baby playthings. That motorized swing may be the last thing that you would have thought of buying, and yet it's the thing that your darling loves the best.

Just be sure to honor your gift-givers with that baby shower. This get-together allows your friends to share in the joy of bringing a new life to earth, as well as recognizing their contributions to your growing family. Because whether you want them to or not, you are having a baby—and people will buy you gifts.

65.

Baby Shower Etiquette

Etiquette is a funny word. The rules of etiquette can mean different things to different people, and generation after generation of families have passed down, as well as revised, these rules. So while the details may have changed over time, the general rules regarding a baby shower are as follows.

Most baby showers are held during the guest of honor's last trimester (usually in month eight or nine). The event is hosted by the mother-to-be's friends or, in some cases, her family.

The pregnant woman's mother, mother-in-law, relatives, close friends, and coworkers may be invited to the celebration. A growing trend has been to forget the "girl" games and include men in the mix. Coed showers are a great way to include all family members.

Another way that showers have changed over the years is that it is now common to throw a shower for a second or even third pregnancy. While these may not be as elaborate as the ones thrown for a first child, they are every bit as helpful to the parents and enjoyable for the guests. In these cases, just like a shower held for a first baby, a baby registry at a designated store or a gift list given to a friend is often utilized to keep track of presents.

In any shower, the mother-to-be has four main duties: 1. Provide the gift registry. 2. Create the guest list and record addresses. 3. Show up at the party. 4. Send out thank-you cards. She does not take on the responsibility of entertaining. Many new moms, in gratitude for all of the attention shown to them, try to take on too much. They want to help plan, prepare food, or even decorate for the shower. This is a job for your friends and family. You are the guest of honor, and one who should be resting, as well!

You will get the opportunity to thank everyone appropriately. No matter how close you may be to your due date, make it a point to build in time to write out your thank-you cards. While much may change in the world of etiquette, the simple courtesy of a thank-you will always be in good taste.

66.

It's Called Transformance

Pregnancy may be filled with particularly complex emotions for some women. It doesn't matter how much you want to hold this precious angel in your arms; once you do so, you are losing a certain amount of freedom. (The freedom to sleep is the first thing that comes to mind.)

There is also the fact that your body is not just for you anymore. Soon, your time won't be yours, either. Also, no matter how committed you may be to growing old with your partner, you are now bound to the man forever.

Additionally, you will be undergoing a change in your identity. First you were you. Then (most likely) you became someone's wife. Now, you are about to become someone's mother. Yup, that will probably be you driving your daughter to school in your bedroom slippers some morning. Perhaps most mornings.

Once your name is officially Mommy, there are no more sick days; no more vacation days; no turning back now. Whatever were you thinking? There may be days that you question your motives in having a child. After all, your life is about to change completely—and chances are that you kind of liked your old life—but change is an important part of life. It's how we learn, how we grow.

This may be the greatest growth spurt that you'll have in your adult life. Becoming a parent is a big responsibility—but it's also one of the greatest joys you will know.

The first time that your baby falls sound asleep in the warmth of your arms, and you catch just a glimpse of your reason for being here on earth, you will understand that change is a good thing. It makes us wiser and teaches us what's important. It's certainly worth a few nights of sleep.

67.

Take Advantage of Childbirth Classes

At some point during your pregnancy, your friends, physician, or midwife will most likely suggest that you enroll in childbirth preparedness classes. Lamaze and Bradley are the two most popular of such classes. However, there are several options available.

The goal of these classes is simply to teach you pain management. Although many women do opt for natural births while using these relaxation tools, the classes themselves may be empowering, regardless of how you intend to deliver your child. In fact, even if you are certain that your delivery will be conducted via a scheduled Cesarean section, childbirth preparedness classes are valuable.

First, the classes counsel you on how to utilize relaxation techniques. These are skills that you can use any time that you are under stress. The myriad techniques often include meditation, creating a comfortable environment, focused breathing, touch, and imagery. Secondly, they will build a stronger bond between you and your birth partner. The classes will also teach you different options for laboring and birthing positions.

Probably the greatest benefit of these classes is the opportunity to meet and form friendships with other prospective parents. Many couples report that they have met some of their closest friends in childbirth classes. They formed relationships with other people who were also experiencing a powerful life change at the same time. These couples found themselves on the phone with each other frequently during pregnancy. "Who else," one new mother reasoned, "could I call for company while eating my midnight snack? Only a pregnant woman is religiously awake and eating at that hour." The friends truly provided support for each other through labor, babyhood, and beyond.

Regardless of how you intend to deliver your baby, childbirth preparedness classes offer many advantages. Pain management, parental preparedness, and solid friendships may be just a few of the reasons to enroll in such a course.

68.

Take the Hospital Tour

It has been said that the greatest fear is the fear of the unknown. Labor is always an "unknown." Even if this is your eleventh child, each labor and delivery are different. If this is your first child, however, you may have a particularly strong fear of the unknown—starting with the environment in which you will perform the most strenuous physical feat of your life.

Just as your caregiver may recommend taking a childbirth preparedness class, he or she will probably also suggest a prenatal tour of the hospital or birthing center in which you plan to give birth. Initially, this may sound like a waste of time. You will, after all, be at that very hospital or center to give birth shortly. Why tour and talk about it beforehand?

There are several reasons. The first is that it may serve as a very strong calming influence during the stress of your labor. Once one of the major unknowns is eliminated, and you have seen the hospital and perhaps met the staff, your emotional state during delivery will be that much more peaceful. The tour will also familiarize you with the different types of rooms that the hospital may have available (some have "suites" large enough for an entire family); the pain medications (such as spinals and epidurals) and how they work; and the surgical room in which a Cesarean may be performed.

One of the most important features of the hospital tour may be the ability to pre-register at the admissions desk (there's nothing worse than timing contractions while trying to remember your social security number) and learning where to check in for childbirth in order to be taken straight to a room. Besides that, you usually get a big bag full of free goodies from the makers of baby products during your hospital tour.

Visiting the place where you plan to deliver your baby takes away half of the anxious unknown feeling. Even if you've given birth in this hospital before, a "refresher course" of what is to come may relax you when the day arrives.

69.

Consider a Doula

Doulas are paid to coach someone to do what millions of women have done for thousands of years. It may sound silly to you, but rest assured, it is not.

For one thing, for thousands of years, women have lived in close proximity to (if not in the same household as) their relatives. They had mom, grandmom, great-grandmom, and twelve sisters in the room to encourage and advise them. They were all there to provide the comfort and protection needed during childbirth. These days, women are not always so lucky to have their mothers around to mother them when they become mothers.

A doula (a Greek word that means "woman caregiver") may be able to provide what no one else can. Doulas give labor support or postpartum home care services. Some provide both. A doula is trained in the emotional, physical, and psychological aspects of childbirth. She can provide comfort in many ways, including back rubs and information regarding your labor. Doulas are by no means medical personnel. However, a doula will facilitate and act as your advocate with your medical staff.

A doula's attention is focused strictly on you, the mother-to-be. She will also assist your husband and friends, if requested to do so by you, but she is there to be your support.

Most doulas will visit prior to the birth to get to know you and learn what your wishes are regarding the birth. Many labor support doulas also stop by after the birth. Of course, postpartum doulas will be there for you when you need help breastfeeding, cleaning up the house, or running errands. Unless you're willing to move back into your mother's house and invite all of your sisters to come join you for the birth, where else can you get treatment like that?

Is hiring a doula considered to be extravagant? Perhaps. Then again, doesn't every woman who is going to give birth deserve to have a strong female companion by her side?

70.

Behold: Your Birth Partner

Chances are that your birth partner will be the father of your baby, but this is not always the situation. More and more single women are opting to become mothers. There is also the possibility that your partner travels extensively or is in the armed services. Then there are those men who turn blue at the sight of blood. If this is the case, it is probably best to designate an alternate birth partner—just in case.

Most men are a little nervous about the whole birthing process. For one thing, they're not really sure how the mechanics of childbirth work. The bigger problem is that men are accustomed to being the "rescuers." If we have a headache, they sweetly bring us an aspirin. If we need to cry, they offer a shoulder. If we have a baby—well, how can they fix that? They often become intimidated by the process, because they believe that we expect them to take away our pain. For some, it's just too difficult to see their most beloved in pain—and not be able to physically help them. This is probably the reason that—not too long ago—most men usually paced the hospital halls in anticipation of the announcement, "You have a daughter" or "You have a son" at which time they would light up the obligatory cigar.

Today's men don't have it quite so easy; nor does any other person appointed as a birth partner. Then again, today's men never had it so good. Our partners get to experience the birth with us. They are allowed to be present in the moment, and they can comfort us in our time of need.

To some people, this may be an intimidating responsibility. If that is the case, designate a backup birthing partner or a doula. A backup or a doula not only relieves your discomforts, but she can also provide relief for the nervous father, because he knows that your comfort is no longer "all up to him."

The main thing is this—be sure that you have confidence in the abilities of whomever you choose to be your birthing partner. Whether that person is your mate, your mother, or your best friend, it will help to know that your own anxiety will be taken care of in that person's hands.

71.

Prepare a Birth Plan

Okay, not everything goes according to a plan. That may be especially true when it comes to delivering a baby. Establishing a birth plan with your partner and doctor prior to going into labor will put you all at ease.

A written birth plan expresses your particular wishes regarding your labor and delivery. It is not a script. Situations may arise where your plan cannot (and should not) be followed. However, barring any extenuating circumstances, a plan allows you to choose your options early and communicates those decisions to your caregiver.

Your birth plan may be simple or detailed. Areas of consideration may include your preferences on the following:

- Atmosphere during labor—dim light/music or peace and quiet
- Mobility and birthing positions
- Those present during birth
- Who cuts the umbilical cord

- Pain relief options
- Use of epidural anesthesia, forceps, or vacuum extraction
- Circumcision (for boys)
- Breastfeeding after birth (also in the delivery room)

Once you and your partner have penned your preferences, make several copies. You will want to discuss your list with your partner and doctor (midwife, nurse practitioner, doula, or personal childbirth coach) around week thirty-four of your pregnancy. Be sure that those people have a copy. Another one should go into your hospital or birthing center chart. Be sure to tuck a third one into your hospital bag.

Again, not everything may go according to plan. At least you'll have the peace of mind of knowing that your preferences are duly noted.

72.

Be Prepared at All Times

Admit it—somewhere in the back of your mind is this image. You wake up the morning of your due date to find that your water has broken in your sleep. You roll over, awaken your partner with a kiss, and tell him that it's time. Everyone dresses, gets organized, has breakfast, and rides to the hospital for a lovely day of childbirth.

It's not going to happen like this.

Very few (if any) women actually give birth on their due dates. In fact, many babies make their entrance into the world a little earlier than expected. That familiar fantasy of rolling over at night and noticing a puddle on one's mattress is more of movie scene than a real-life occurrence. Most of the time when one's water breaks, it is more of a trickle than a gush. Additionally, nearly half of all women actually have their water broken by their caregiver during birth.

It helps to be prepared. Keep your insurance card in your wallet. Carry your caregiver's phone number with you at all times. Do the same for the contact numbers of your birth coach, your partner, doula, and mother or father. Install an infant seat in your car. (You are not allowed to leave the hospital without one.) Pack your bag, plan your trip to the hospital, and set up your nursery.

Remember that you truly could go into labor at any moment, and while most labors do last for hours, there are those stories out there of women who labored for twenty-five minutes before the baby's head was crowning. These women practically walked into the hospital with a baby dangling between their knees.

Who knows? You might just be one of the lucky ones. One minute you're at the office preparing a speech, and the next minute you become a new mother. Push, plop, you're done. No mattress puddles. No breakfast.

It will help to be prepared. Once you hit your third trimester, the moment could be now.

73.

Don't Skip the Practice Drill

Unless you work at the hospital or birth center where you intend to deliver your child, or you are planning a home birth, it is a really good idea to make a practice drive to the hospital. This is not a silly, time-wasting exercise. It is a step that can prepare you in many ways for the important trip.

Even if you have been to the building numerous times, things can change. Roads are sometimes under construction. New traffic lights or lane shifts might not be noticed by a nervous father-to-be. Where exactly is the admissions desk? Find out during your test run.

If you take the hospital tour, it can double as your practice drill. Be sure to take the route that you are most comfortable on. Avoid the highway if speed makes you anxious or the back roads if stop signs drive you crazy. Either way, it is a good idea to put a map in the glove compartment, just in case there's an obstruction that you need to go around. More than one woman, for example, has gone into labor during a holiday parade.

Be sure to note the approximate amount of time that it takes to get there—which will inevitably feel like hours when the big day comes. The drive may feel like it takes even longer for your partner, who will most likely be behind the wheel.

Women have pregnancy nightmares that they've left their babies somewhere; men have haunting fears that women will deliver their children in the car on the way to the hospital. They worry that they'll have to pull over, find some water to boil, and coach the women through labor in the backseat of the family wagon. A practice drive to the hospital or birthing center can help to ease your anxiety when the time arrives. It will familiarize you with the route, narrow down your timetable, and give your partner a chance to scout out areas where he can pull off the road, find some water to boil, and deliver the baby.

74.

Get Your Bag Together

Most pregnant women pack their hospital bags far in advance of their due date. Why not? Looking at that bag by the door reminds you that someday soon, those swollen ankles, backaches, and exhausted days will be a thing of the past. (Well, maybe not the exhausted days!) It will also be the day that you anticipate—holding the new love of your life in your arms. That means that you also need to pack for the little one.

Packing an overnight bag for someone you haven't met yet will feel surreal. It will also feel rewarding. Be sure that you have everything that you need for your first nights together.

For You
- Telephone list
- Copy of birth plan
- Camera and extra film
- Snacks and drinks for you, your partner, and family

- Candles, music, or other focal-point items
- Favorite pillow
- Pajamas
- Extra socks and slippers
- Large, comfortable going-home outfit
- Nursing bra and large panties
- Pen and paper
- Reading material
- Makeup case (You'll want a little lipstick on for all of those photos.)

For Baby
- T-shirt
- Socks
- Blanket
- Burping cloth
- Outfit and/or pajamas

Once your bag is packed and ready to go, it's one more thing that you can check off your "to-do" list. That will help you to feel another degree calmer when the day arrives. Having your bag together might even eliminate some of those pregnancy dreams in which you're giving birth while wearing a cocktail dress and heels.

75.

Relish Your Relationship with Your Partner

If you and your partner are married, you became a family the moment you both said the words "I do." Now, however, you are about to become a very different type of family. All of your friends are right. Children change everything. Both you and your partner will be more focused on this tiny little being than you are on yourselves or each other. That is why it is important to put aside some quiet time now to simply enjoy your relationship and focus on each other while you still can.

In the first trimester, why not evaluate the goals that you both have as individuals, as a couple, and as a family? The path to those goals may change somewhat while you are chasing around the pitter-patter of tiny feet, but your dreams themselves will still be important—even if they are delayed. Is there, for example, still a way for you to take night courses after you have a new baby? Can he continue to build his own business with the demands of fatherhood? What about where you live? If you have been talking about making a physical move, this may be the time to take action. Moving while nine months pregnant, or with a newborn, can feel like it is ten times the amount of work.

The second trimester lends itself quite nicely to a great getaway with your guy. It doesn't need to be a month in the Canary Islands (although if you can do it, go for it). Even a hop in the car to a nearby weekend resort will give you a chance to reconnect with your honey. This mid-pregnancy stage is when most women feel their best. The morning sickness is behind them. The swollen ankles are yet to come. Some women, in fact, gain energy midway through their pregnancies. Since travel is not yet restricted, this may be the last opportunity that you get for the next few years to steal your partner away for some time alone. Why not take advantage of it?

The final stretch of pregnancy is a great time to make dates to enjoy the local art exhibits, movies, and restaurants that you have wanted to check out. Now, it's fairly easy. Toss on your maternity dress and a little lipstick and go. Soon, you'll need to collect three hundred items to stuff into a diaper bag before you stroll the baby to the car and strap him or her into the car seat—only to realize that you have spit all over your shirt and need to go back inside and change your clothes.

Take advantage of this time to enjoy your mate and your freedom. Remember to relish your relationship.

76.

Enjoy Nesting

Throughout a woman's pregnancy, she may find herself sticking close to home more than usual. She may clean her house more often, decide to redecorate a room, or want fresh flowers in her kitchen at all times. This is called the "nesting instinct."

Nesting also affects fathers-to-be. He may suddenly repair all of the items that have been building up on his workbench for a year. He might get the urge to reseed the lawn—every week. Some men even take an interest in cooking or figure out how the washing machine works.

Enjoy your nesting instincts. It's your psyche's way of making your home into a new kind of home. You are now preparing for an addition to your family. If this is your first child, it may very well transform you and your partner into a family. You are paving the way for a new life ahead of you.

Toward the end of your pregnancy, the word "nesting" may take on an even stronger meaning. The organizing and beautifying of your home may go beyond normal behavior. Some women find themselves dusting every window frame and doorsill that they can reach. Others scrub the refrigerator out on a daily basis. Some have installed fire extinguishers in every room of the house, while others wander around applying Wite-Out to every chip or mark in the white paint on their walls. There is no limit to the nesting instinct of some moms-to-be.

Your actions may seem a bit outlandish, but this is just nature's way of having some good, wholesome fun. Relax, and let your urges go. After all, won't it feel good to have that refrigerator (finally!) scrubbed clean?

77.

Create Space for the New Family Member

I f you have the space, money, and decorating acumen to create a picture-perfect nursery, then by all means, study the magazines and have a blast. Many of us, however, need a little help with the nursery. For example, what if there is no separate room available for baby? For the first few months, the baby will probably sleep in a bassinet in your room. This is the most convenient way for groggy parents to respond to all-night feedings.

While the bassinet may remain in the bedroom, there needs to be a space for the baby's crib. The baby will need drawers to store clothes, and a diaper-changing station is an important designation. Although some women claim that they can change their child's diaper anywhere with a well-stocked diaper bag, most of us prefer to have a designated diaper-changing station in our homes. It just seems much easier to keep all of those diapers, wipes, ointments, and lotions in one space. Additionally, a diaper bin next to the station is essential.

You may be surprised at how quickly the baby outgrows that cute bassinet. Eventually, you will want to have a space for your little one—if not just for the baby, then for all of the stuff that is required to care for him or her. The good news is that babies do not need large rooms—but they do need some room. A nook or cranny will do for a while, as long as it is designated baby space.

As your baby grows, he or she can be slowly relocated into another room. If you have no spare space in your current home, however, you may need to start looking for larger quarters once the baby arrives. Your newborn may someday be bunking with a younger sibling.

Remember that for the next few months, your own special space in the house will probably be the most comfortable chair. This will be where you end up feeding your newborn a lot of the time. Perhaps you should move the chair to a quieter room. Place a small table next to the chair for books, magazines, extra cloths, and glasses of water, and be sure to add extra pillows for comfort. That big comfy chair may become your favorite place to be to share the first months of life with your baby.

78.

Stock Up on Baby's Basic Needs

Babies need a lot of stuff. That is a fact. However, advertisements and marketing may lead couples to believe that babies need even more stuff than they do. Here are the basics of what you will need to care for your newborn (aside from love, but the baby will already have that).

- Diaper bag—Be sure that it is roomy enough to carry four diapers, burping cloths, a change of clothes, bottles (if bottle-feeding), bottled water and snacks for Mom, rattles, toys, and your own purse, which you will inevitably try to toss into the larger bag.

- Diapers—Whether you prefer cloth or disposable, stock up well in advance of the baby's birth. The last thing that you want to do in the first few days after delivery is run out for diapers.

- Bathing gel, diaper rash ointment, petroleum jelly, cotton swabs (to clean the umbilical cord), nasal aspirator, and thermometer

- T-shirts, socks (at least five pairs), outfits, pajamas, and hats for the baby—Babies go through a lot of clothing changes. They also outgrow their clothes very quickly. Six outfits and sets of pajamas for you should be enough until you can do the laundry—every couple of days.

- Bottles and breast pump or formula. If you plan to breastfeed, this can wait a while. If you are doing a combination of both or bottle-feeding, start with six bottles and two large packages of formula.

- Linens, which include burping cloths (a dozen), receiving blankets (at least five), bibs, and bassinet and crib sheets

Stock up on your baby's basic needs now. In this way, you will ensure a smooth arrival when you bring your little one to live in his or her new home.

79.

Breast or Bottle?

Whether you choose to nurse your baby or bottle-feed is your own decision. It's a highly personal decision, and it needs to be based on your own lifestyle.

There are several health benefits to nursing, and in many ways, nursing can be easier than the alternative. There are no bottles to wash or expensive formula. There is no warming up milk at three in the morning. Just snuggle your baby and doze off.

Additionally, nursing feels good. In fact, it can be a transcendent experience, resulting in one very satisfied mom and one extremely happy baby. This may also create a stronger bond between you and your child.

Finally, breastfeeding helps to shrink your uterus back to its pre-pregnancy size. Each contraction that you experience while nursing is actually your womb becoming its former self again.

On the other hand, there are advantages to bottle-feeding. You know how much your baby is eating. Daddy can also bond with baby by sharing the feedings. You don't need to hide yourself in public when it's baby's feeding time.

With bottle-feeding, your baby won't be affected by any medications that you need to take or by that glass of wine that you've waited nine months to drink. Your food choices will not be limited, and you can probably incorporate more of your own life into motherhood than if you were exclusively nursing.

Some women manage to get the best of both worlds with a combination of breast- and bottle-feeding. Others prefer to stick with one method or the other. Whichever way you choose to feed your child, do not let anyone pressure you into a decision. Ignore your aunt who tells you that all worthy mothers breastfeed until their children are five years old. Turn a deaf ear to your boss when she states that no self-respecting businesswoman would even consider breastfeeding her child.

Do what feels right. Do what is best for you. It is, after all, your decision.

80.

Plan to Remember the Moment

By your third trimester, the pregnancy thing is probably getting old. In fact, you may feel as though you've been pregnant ever since you can remember and will remain pregnant for the rest of your life.

Even though the days may seem endless, the time itself is fleeting. Someday, you may want something other than a moth-eaten maternity dress to help you remember these magical days of creating your child inside your womb. Why not immortalize these days by keeping a journal, having tasteful photographs taken, or even getting a belly-mold?

A journal may be the best way to remember the ins and outs of pregnancy. While writing your life's notes, you may believe that you will read the book a hundred times—or you may never expect to read it again. Either way, you will dig it out and read it with great interest the moment that your own daughter or daughter-in-law announces that she is pregnant with your first grandchild.

Many women opt to have photos taken of their fully pregnant silhouette. This is not something to be shy about. No matter how "fat" you may feel at this moment (especially in your third trimester), you will soon be wearing your favorite blue jeans again and wishing you had a photo of your child-bearing days. You may be as fully clothed or tastefully unclothed as you please. Professional photos are always a treat. However, do not put off the project just because you feel a little shy about disrobing in front of strangers. Tossing on a sarong and thrusting a disposable camera into your sweetie's hand as you pull him into the backyard for some shots will still serve as a reminder of how you looked in your "pregnant state."

Belly-molds (papier-mâché, clay, or cast-iron replicas of your pregnant self) or commissioned sculptures and portraits are other ways to pay homage to your gestation days. Why not indulge in a work of art that celebrates the beauty of pregnancy?

While these days may feel never-ending, they will be over sooner than you expect. You deserve to give yourself the beautiful gift of remembering the moment.

81.

Keep Your Expectations in Check

Thanks to the advanced state of prenatal care, you can rest assured that your baby will most likely be born healthy, with all ten fingers and toes. Beyond that, you may dream that your child will inherit your curly blond hair and your husband's blue eyes. Be careful not to allow your expectations to control your emotions.

Your baby will be beautiful, no matter what he or she physically looks like. Yes, he might end up with Uncle Tom's nose. She may have inherited Grandma's recessed hairline. That won't matter one bit. Your darling will be the most beautiful baby that you've ever laid eyes on.

Other expectations that we secretly covet about our children include disposition, intelligence, and talents. We all come to realize that no matter how calm and poised we may (or may not) be, our children can turn out to be just the opposite. They all have their own sweet personalities.

The same goes for talent. Even if both you and your partner are musically inclined, there is no guarantee that your baby will turn into the world's next Liberace.

Probably the biggest expectations we hold are for ourselves. No, we will not be perfect mothers. There is no such thing. Yes, we will make mistakes. Everyone does. Okay, there will be questions—a lot of questions. At first, breastfeeding may be a challenge. You won't know the difference between a hungry cry and a tired cry. (No one does.) It may take a few tries before you figure out how the car seat works.

You'll get it. Just give yourself some time—and remember to keep your expectations in check.

82.

Set Yourself Up

A newborn baby can cause you to feel love on many different levels that you've never felt before. You will find yourself spending hours just standing over the infant's crib, staring at the beautiful being that you brought into this world.

A newborn baby can also cause you to feel exhaustion on many different levels that you've never felt before. Add in a little disorientation, a lot of forgetfulness, and a dull achy feeling in your bones from having given birth. There are a few things that you can do right now to make your life easier over the next few months.

Talk to your partner. Let him know how much your workload has increased—you have now added the exhaustion of giving birth and taking care of a newborn to your life. You know that he already plans to help, but you will feel better to hear that reassurance.

Get your house in order. Repair any major appliances now. Make it a point to keep up with your laundry and day-to-day organizing. Once baby is born, you won't have time to play catch-up.

Either write out your bills ahead of time or write out a bill schedule. In the excitement of having a baby, it is surprisingly common that people forget about their bills. Similarly, address your baby announcement envelopes. Remember to stock up on stamps.

Buy nonperishables in bulk. That includes diapers and diaper wipes, paper products, canned foods, and cereals. The fewer trips you need to make to the store after delivery, the better.

Line up help. Your mother, mother-in-law, sister, and friends may all offer to come help with the new baby. Let them!

Plan your meals. In your last trimester, make doubles of your favorite recipes and freeze them for quick meals with a newborn. Another (not as nutritious) option is to take a walk down the frozen food aisle of your favorite grocery store and try out some new, easy-to-cook ideas.

Choose a pediatrician. Well-baby visits start at the age of two weeks. Start soliciting your friends' advice, and decide on a pediatrician before you give birth. Those first two weeks fly by very quickly.

You are making the biggest day-by-day (sometimes minute-by-minute) adjustment of your life. You'll be thankful that some of your potential tasks have already been completed.

83.

Take Control of Your Labor Fears

You can't wait to see your angel. You may also be a little nervous at the whole process of delivering the baby. After all, the baby coming out is much larger than the tiny embryo that first signaled life beginning within you. It can be a scary thought.

It doesn't help that every woman you met for the last nine months had a delivery horror story to tell you about. Aside from the truly chilling cases when someone (mother or baby) nearly didn't make it, many stories sound worse than they are.

For example, when your Aunt Edna announces that she went through seventy-two hours of labor, only to have a Cesarean section in the end, every woman in the room might cringe. However, Edna didn't really elaborate on the details. If she had, you would know that her contractions started Tuesday morning at ten and ended around noon. She had another three contractions Wednesday night. (In her mind, she was "still" in labor.) By Thursday morning, she had three straight hours of contractions and went to the hospital for the

Cesarean section that she and her doctor had already agreed upon due to the baby's breeched position.

To keep in step, you will most likely have your own delivery horror story once your baby is born. There are surprises around every corner. Some women go into labor while attending football games. Others catch a cold on their due date. Many more drive to the hospital, only to be sent home, and then they drive back again the same day.

Whatever happens during your delivery, you can trust that it will sound scarier much later when you tell the story than it truly is at the time. By then, you will have earned the right to tell the story any which way you desire!

84.

To Medicate or Not to Medicate

Unless one needs to have a Cesarean section, the question of whether or not to accept pain medication is one that most women consider at great length. Childbirth doesn't come easily, and pain relief is an important consideration.

A natural birth does create a more intense memory for Mom without any potential side effects for the baby. Then again, many pregnant women have toddled into the hospital claiming that they want a drug-free birth, only to be screaming for medication once they have reached around six centimeters dilation. In fact, over eighty percent of all birthing moms today use some type of pain medication. Roughly fifty percent of these women had planned on using all-natural relief when they walked through the hospital doors.

Not everyone uses medication, but it is important to discuss your pain relief options with your doctor or midwife. In general, there are three types of pain relief available.

Natural pain relief can be anything that makes a laboring woman feel more relaxed and comfortable. It can include support from the birth partner, visualization, yoga, walking, hypnosis, acupuncture, acupressure, position changes, water, and massage.

Narcotics are drugs, such as Demerol and Stadol, which are injected into a vein or muscle to dull labor pain. They tend to make mothers and babies sleepy and are therefore mostly used in early labor to help women rest and conserve energy.

An epidural—also called regional anesthesia or spinal anesthesia—is the most common form of pain relief in the United States. An epidural catheter is inserted into the back and delivers the medication as needed. Most patients feel nothing below the waist. It can be used for a vaginal birth or Cesarean section.

Each of the painkillers has benefits and drawbacks. Again, be sure to familiarize yourself with the pain relief medications prior to delivery. Even if you do not plan to use medication, you may just fall into the category of the fifty percent who change their mind in the end.

85.

Who Will Witness the Birth?

The birth of a new baby is a family experience. Quite often, your family will show up at your bedside with popcorn in their hands, expecting a front row seat to the event.

You will save yourself a lot of stress during your labor if you clarify who you want to have with you when you actually deliver your baby. Your father-in-law, for example, might automatically think that he's invited when he is the last person that you want to be viewing your anatomy. It's best if everyone understands the rules from the beginning.

Obviously, if you give birth by Cesarean section, your options are limited. Most hospitals allow only one person (if anyone) to view the procedure. The person who does will—in some ways—get to know your body better than you do—from the inside out.

Cesarean sections are sometimes required at the last minute. Take a moment now to talk to your partner (and your birth partner if they're not the same person) about their position on being in the operating room. Since you will most likely be awake, and not able to see the surgery via a curtain between you and your belly, it is comforting to have a friend in the room with you. If the friend, however, is someone who becomes queasy at the sight of blood, he or she will not be very much comfort. Consider leaving such a person on the outside of the operating room door.

In most cases, a vaginal delivery is performed, and today's birthing suites are large enough to accommodate your entire family, neighbors, the postman, and the family pet. Many suites do have the ability to place your family and friends near your shoulders, where they do not have an actual view of the delivery.

Think about how comfortable you'll feel with spectators. Witnessing a birth is a magical experience. A lot of people may want to share this moment. It's up to you to decide (beforehand, since you will not be clearheaded when you are dilated by seven centimeters) whom you believe should or should not be in the room. Remember that in the end, it is still your body.

86.

Smile for the Camera—or Not

You have waited nine (or perhaps more) months for this event. This will be the only birth of your child. Why wouldn't you want to capture the moment any way you can—including on a videotape? Well, you may want to do that—or you may not.

The first thing to think about is your own modesty level. A full view of the birth is not necessarily something that you will want to show at your child's sixteenth birthday party. (It may not be something that your child will want you to show at any time.) You may, at the very least, opt for an over-the-shoulder angle for the camera. Be sure that the cameraperson knows your wishes on this issue.

Another thing to consider when it comes to videotaping a birth is that the pain and negative aspects of delivery—like all things—will fade with time. A tape, however, will serve as a photograph of the experience. In other words, all of that huffing and puffing will be immortalized—as well as all that screaming you may do at your doctor or partner while the baby is crowning. (You'll be angry at everyone by the time you have dilated to ten centimeters—except for your anesthesiologist, if you choose to use painkillers.)

On the other hand, a video may be a sentimental reminder of the day that you brought your sweet angel into this world. Two months from now, you will barely remember what the baby looked like on the day that he or she was born. A videotape is a beautiful keepsake.

Whether or not you choose to have the delivery videotaped is a highly personal decision. If you have a Cesarean section, you will need to check with your physician to see if videotaping is permitted.

Whichever way you give birth, if you have a videographer present, make sure that he or she isn't the type who faints at the sight of blood. No one appreciates a shot of the hospital floor.

87.

Check Out Child Care Now

You may be lucky enough to have one or both sets of grandparents living close by who will gladly watch their newest grandchild while you work or rest. You may even have sisters, brothers, aunts, and close friends who are thrilled at the idea of babysitting. Enjoy this, and take advantage of it.

However, many couples will need to find someone whom they trust to take care of the most precious thing in their lives. Whether you need to locate daycare while you go back to work or a sitter while you get some relief, start now. You'll be glad that you did.

The first day that you leave your newborn alone with the "nanny," you will start to question your decision. Did you do the right thing? Is the sitter trustworthy? You may find yourself loitering around outside for a while before you peek through the window to make sure that your little one is okay. This will be true whether or not the nanny is a daycare worker, full-time nanny, part-time babysitter, or your own mother.

As with most important decisions, your best bet may be asking friends and coworkers for recommendations. This is especially important if you need to choose daycare. Start now. Many centers have waiting lists. If you need to go back to work after your maternity leave, do not wait until the baby is born to find daycare. Now is when you have the time. At least narrow your search down to two or three nearby centers.

Stop by. Observe the children at play. Make sure that the facility is clean and childproofed. Watch how the staff interacts with the children when playing and when disciplining them. Then stop by again—unannounced. Make sure that you are comfortable with your choice. Ask questions—a lot of them. Get credentials. Be a bit of a pest.

In the end, you will be the one who can breathe easier knowing that your child is in safe hands. Well, maybe you'll breathe just a little easier. Remember, as a mother, you are fully entitled to peek in the windows anytime you like.

88.

Ask for Help with the Housework

Traditionally, and still today, the majority of the housework falls on a woman's shoulders. Since the average man around the house does not dedicate as much time and energy toward cleaning, he really doesn't realize what is involved in the process. Don't expect him to know what needs to be done. Ask for help for specific tasks. It may seem obvious to you that a woman who cannot reach her own ankles cannot possibly scrub the bathtub. Believe it or not, the thought never has occurred to him.

Unfortunately, women usually need to ask for help with the housework. He may be eager to help you with your pregnancy—he just doesn't know how. Let him know how he can be of assistance. Tell him that the laundry basket is too heavy for your back—and since he's taking it to the washer, maybe he could sort through the darks and toss a load in.

Similarly, your well-meaning friends and family often don't think of housework as a way to help, so when they call and ask, "Is there anything I can do to help?" don't be shy. Try, "You know, I've always loved your cooking. Maybe you could come over one night, and we'll write up a grocery list, go to the store, and cook for a couple of hours. That way, we'll be set up when the baby is born." Your friend who loves to cook will love the compliment and the evening, and you will end up with some great—and unique—meals in your freezer for when you need them.

You can ask for help with other tasks, as well. People are usually happy to stop by the dry cleaners, pick up a few things from the grocery store, or baby-sit your other children for a while when you are pregnant. All you need to do is ask.

89.

Make Your Health a Priority

For nine months, you've been watching what you eat and drink, avoiding some of your favorite foods, and exercising moderately, and you may have had to give up smoking, caffeine, and alcohol. You've done your duty, right?

Not quite. The grand finale is right around the corner. You've done your best to protect your unborn child. Now it's time to protect yourself. Labor is the most physically grueling thing that most women will undertake. Yes, it's a natural part of life. Yes, trillions of women before you have given birth. That doesn't mean that it doesn't take its toll.

From now on, you need to focus on preparing your body for this event. Preparing simply means making sure that you are physically ready. Eat well (as well as you can, despite the fact that you are craving all sorts of junk food). Rest often. Keep taking those prenatal vitamins. Most importantly, listen to your body's cues.

Some women find that exercise or meditation gives them the ability to listen to their own bodies. Try taking long walks, meditating, or enrolling in a prenatal yoga class. (Do not do any of these things without your physician's approval.)

Through exercise and meditation, you can start to connect with your own body. You can listen to positive and negative feelings and find new and efficient ways to respond to them. This will be especially helpful as you near your delivery date and begin experiencing new and different aches and pains.

Sometimes, people need to find a way to listen to their bodies, and pregnancy is one such time. The best way to do this is to keep your body as healthy and rested as possible and be mindful of how you respond to it.

90.

"This Is Taking Forever!"

At some point, it will feel as though every relative and friend tells you a story about giving birth after month seven when they didn't suspect a thing—and a few women do give birth to perfectly healthy babies a month before their due dates. It might make you suspect something—in fact, it may make you wake up every day around month seven and wonder, "Is today the day?" The hospital bag is packed. Childbirth classes have ended. Friends have started to call every couple of days. What if you burst before the baby shower—or during the baby shower?

The wait has begun. You're nowhere near your due date—but you're anticipating labor at any moment. This situation gets old very quickly. In fact, many women start to wonder if they'll *ever* give birth—and they're only at month eight! The fact is that over half of all women deliver their first child *later* than the due date.

It may be discouraging, but there is a good side to waiting. Right now, your body is putting the finishing touches on your child.

For one thing, your body begins to supply the baby with antibodies through the placenta. These antibodies will help your child's immune system fight infection for the first six months of life. Your baby's body is also producing a surge of fetal hormones that may help with the maintenance of blood pressure and blood sugar levels after birth. Probably the most important things that happen during the last couple weeks of pregnancy are the development of your baby's lungs and brain. These are the last two organs to fully develop and two of the most vital to your baby's survival.

Why not give your baby as much time as he or she needs? That way, the baby will come out as smart and healthy as possible. It's only another day in your life, but it could mean a world of difference to your child.

91.

Including Your Other Children

The birth of a new baby is an exciting event for every member of the family. It can also be a time of fear and vulnerability for your other children. They may feel that they are going to be "replaced" by the newest kid—and in a way, they will be.

No matter how well you balance your family, a new baby needs to be the focus of your time and attention for a while. Help your other children understand this by making them part of the birthing experience and easing them into their older sibling roles.

First, prepare them for the birth. From the moment that you tell them that you are expecting another child, also tell them exactly how far along you are and when your due date is. Remember that kids are more oriented toward graphics. Mark your due date on a calendar. Show them the ultrasound print, or point out an image of a fetus at a similar age in a book or on a Web site.

Let your children help you shop for special baby items (including toys and clothes), and tell them what is to be expected during the actual delivery of their sibling. When the day comes, it is up to you to decide if you want to bring your children to the hospital or leave them with relatives. Either way, let them know that they are involved. Phone them often with updates, and have them visit as soon as possible.

You may want your other children to actually to view the birth (either from a full view or an over-the-shoulder position). If so, coach them on the stages of labor beforehand. Since younger ones may become upset by Mommy's discomfort, be sure to have someone in the room (other than your birth partner) available to help support them.

Whether your children are included by phone or in person, make sure that they feel they are part of the birth of their new sibling. Let them put on the baby's first pair of booties or hand the child his or her first rattle. That will help them to ease into their transit as the older children, which will help them to understand the baby's demands.

92.

Expect False Labor

Every first-time mother has the same question: How will I know when I go into labor? Unfortunately, the answer is that sometimes you won't know.

Your earliest contractions might be Braxton Hicks contractions, named for the nineteenth-century English doctor, John Braxton Hicks, who first "discovered" them. Braxton Hicks contractions, a periodic tightening of the uterus, happen from very early on in pregnancy. Most women do not really notice them until the second half of pregnancy. In the third trimester, they can be truly as painful as real labor. Sometimes, it is difficult to distinguish between Braxton Hicks contractions and real labor, which is the reason that these contractions are also called "false labor."

Actually, there is no such thing as false labor. Early contractions are still contractions. They are preparing your body for delivery. Whether your cervix dilates or not, your body has still "gone into labor" for the moment. It may be hours, days, or weeks before you hit "productive labor." That simply means that your cervix is now dilating. Your body has done its job. All of those early contractions did what they were supposed to do, and you're that much closer to delivering your baby.

How will you know the difference? You really don't, at first. There are many experienced moms out there who drove to the hospital intending to deliver their second (or third or fourth) child, only to be sent home. If it happens to you, don't be embarrassed. Your caregiver will prefer the "better-safe-than-sorry" attitude.

Braxton Hicks contractions can certainly feel like the real thing. The trick is consistency. So-called "false labor" may last a minute or an hour, but it stops. Real labor may stop briefly, but it starts right back up. Another thing that can tip you off to Braxton Hicks is that the contractions will stop once you change position (for instance, if you sit down after you've been standing for a while).

If you can't tell the difference between real and false labor, you're in good company. Those early contractions have fooled a lot of women—even women who have been through labor many times in the past.

93.

Ease into Real Labor

Here it is, the moment that you've been awaiting for nine months. You're in labor. It's real. It's regular. The contractions are getting closer and closer together. At this point, there is only one thing that you can do. Relax!

Very few mothers are lucky enough to be in that "I gave birth in thirty-two minutes" category. Most of our bodies need preparation. In fact, the majority of women report that they were in labor for at least two to four hours before it was diagnosed. That is because most often, labor pains start as tight cramps every twenty to thirty minutes. Pregnant women experience a lot of cramps—"Is this labor? Are these just more cramps?"—so they keep shopping.

Eventually, the cramps increase. You're now doubled over every fifteen minutes. Still, it's not a great enough sensation to interrupt your supper (for too long). However, after a couple of hours, you begin to believe that you are in labor.

Now what? Now, relax and conserve your energy. Many, many women have spent hours in this state. You could spend from two to twenty hours in "light labor" before your physician or midwife will attend to you. Medical books claim that the average amount of time spent in labor for a first child is twelve hours, but every birth is different.

This is the time to enjoy what is happening in your own body and ease into labor. Put on a good movie. Plan a celebratory (but light) meal. Start reading that book that you plan to engage yourself in (thereby focusing on anything other than the contractions) while you are in labor.

Enjoy this time. Take it gently, and make the most of it. Honor your body now, and it will thank you when it comes time to deliver your baby.

94.

Make Friends with Your Nurses

Even the meekest, most mild-mannered women have been known to turn into raving maniacs during the delivery of a child. Blame it on hormones. Blame it on pain. Blame it on your partner—he's the one who got you into this situation in the first place, right? You may even find yourself screaming at your midwife or your doctor. Don't be too concerned if you do this. They have witnessed labor in the past, and they usually don't take it personally. It's considered just another occupational hazard.

Some women have even confessed to cursing their mothers (for not telling the truth about the pain of childbirth) or their birth partners (just because the Lamaze teacher said that they might). However, if you are laboring in a hospital or a birthing center, there is one person you should try very hard not to yell at—and that is your delivery nurse. In fact, it's a good idea to try to make friends with all of the nurses who care for you.

Your delivery nurse, in particular, will become your best friend during your labor and the birth of your child (especially if you do not have a doula present). She's the one you will depend on for those coveted ice chips. She understands what all of blips and bleeps from the machines mean. She'll become the one that you trust the most when she says that you're doing "just fine." She may be the one who takes your baby's first photo. She'll also be the one who whisks your baby away for tests. As you can see, there are many reasons to be your sweetest self to this person.

Similarly, the nurses who take care of you—and your precious baby—after the birth may become your personal angels of mercy. They are the ones who will comfort you when you are exhausted and every muscle is screaming. They will accompany you on your first post-birth walk, and they will bring all of the ice packs that you need.

More importantly, these are the people who will teach you to breastfeed, clean your baby's umbilical cord scab, and answer all of those questions that will suddenly pop into your head two minutes after you give birth. So make friends with the nurses. Treat them well, and appreciate all of their good help.

95.

Let Go of Cesarean Section Fears

Prior to giving birth, you may find yourself worried that, like so many women before you, you plan to push your child out naturally and end up delivering by Cesarean section. Yes, in some cases, it does happen. In fact, in one of every five cases, it happens. It may even happen in your case.

Be sure to talk to your health care provider regarding his or her position on performing Cesarean sections. It may be, for instance, that the hospital's policy requires a Cesarean section on all full-breech presentations (meaning that the baby's buttocks or feet are facing downward). Your caregiver may also prefer to attempt a breech delivery prior to submitting to surgery. Do take comfort in the fact that most of today's doctors and hospitals will only deliver a child by C-section if it is necessary to ensure the health of the mother or child.

Yes, it can be disappointing to hear those words, "We need to consider a Cesarean section." Your dreams of labor and delivery mostly likely include a final push—not a surgical procedure. If you do hear those words, understand that there is nothing more that you could have done to make a difference. This is absolutely in no way a sign that you have "failed" at childbirth. A successful birth means a healthy baby and a healthy mother.

Some women claim that a Cesarean section "robbed" them of the whole organic childbirth experience. Ask those same women what might have happened if they had attempted a vaginal delivery. While no one really knows the "what ifs" of life with any certainty, those women's physicians determined that vaginal births might have "robbed" the mothers or children of their own health. Then ask yourself what you would rather be robbed of—an organic delivery or a healthy child?

You and your baby may not experience the full slide down the birth canal, but in the end, you will both be safe. When the time comes, that's all that really matters.

96.

Rejoice in Bringing the Baby Home

For nine to ten months, you've been waiting for the day you can bring your darling baby home. It's the first time the child will see the house—the room, the crib, the toys. It is the thrilling beginning of a new life for all of you. You will always remember this day and this house. Take a deep breath and rejoice in this precious moment—and try to fight back the terror!

It will suddenly occur to you that you are now responsible for this tiny, fragile being. If this is your first child, you may be wondering how it is possible that the hospital just let you leave with this baby in your arms. You don't know what you're doing!

There will be no nurses around to help your baby latch onto your breast or bottle. Unless a relative or friend is staying with you the first few days, there will also be no one to change the diapers for you—you'll need to figure out which side is the front all on your own. When your little angel cries, it will be up to you (and Daddy, who may get flustered and hand the baby back to you) to figure out why and how to fix it. It may sound scary. You've probably had more training on taking care of your pets than you've had on caring for a child.

Relax. As intimidating as it may seem, you will sense your way through it. Each day, you'll learn a little bit more, and by the time that second or third child comes around you'll be a professional.

Even then, however, you may make mistakes. Every one of us makes a few parenting mistakes along the way. Honestly, your child will not suffer any long-term damage if it takes a few tries before breastfeeding goes smoothly or if he or she cries for a full ten minutes before you manage to get that burp up.

Enjoy this new beginning. Shrug off your fears that you might not be a good mother. You'll be a terrific mother. Rejoice when it comes time to bring your darling home. (By the way, that little design on the diaper marks the front.)

97.

Birth Announcements

While your closest friends and family members may have already visited you in the hospital or been at your doorstep when you returned home, there will be many others who are eagerly anticipating the birth of your child. Your coworkers, neighbors, and out-of-town friends and relatives will all want to see the adorable new baby you have created. Birth announcements may be in order.

There are two tricks to sending out birth announcements. First, keep it simple. If you have already purchased your announcements and addressed (and stamped) your envelopes while you were pregnant, you will be much more likely to actually send them. Simply fill in the statistics, have Daddy print or order copies of baby's photo, and toss them in the mailbox.

Second, ask for help. Some men are perfectly willing to address envelopes or have pictures printed. Many men will want to be "technologically correct" by sending e-mail announcements. E-mail announcements, by the way, are not such a bad idea as long as all of the important recipients have access to an e-mail address and color printer. If they do not, then your own parents may miss having a tangible photograph of their newest grandchild to show off to their coworkers and golf buddies. This means that you may end up doing it both ways anyway, and that doesn't make things any easier.

Your best bet may be to delegate the photo duties to Dad and enlist the help of a girlfriend for all of the other detail work. Plan to spend a couple of hours with your friend to take turns addressing, stamping, and swaying baby. Keep it simple. Get it done at one time. Let your loved ones share in your joy.

98.

Honor Your Body's Need to Rest

Why is it that we have been conditioned to believe that we must dedicate nine months toward creating a child, deliver a healthy baby, and then make it downtown for our hair appointment at noon the next day? Most of us probably could accomplish it, but think of everything that your body has been through. Why would you want to push yourself at this time?

Taking care of a newborn is a huge responsibility, and your body is fatigued. You need your rest.

There is a reason that your doctor tells you that you need to take it easy and not to lift anything heavier than your baby for the next six weeks. Labor is quite a feat, and your body is now recovering physically from the birth—not to mention that you are adjusting to your new role of motherhood, and changes of this magnitude take a lot of energy.

The old adage to sleep when baby sleeps is the best advice out there. Forget the dust in the living room. Ignore the laundry. Eat what is nutritious and easy to toss together. Hopefully, you'll have a freezer full of prepared meals. If not, be sure to send your partner to the store for nutritious snacks and quick meal ingredients. Do not count on him to do the cooking and cleaning. You will find that his help is much more valuable when it comes to rocking the baby so that you can catch a few minutes of shuteye.

One hundred years ago, women were not allowed out of bed for a month after giving birth. There may be some wisdom in that practice. Even if you feel great, you are probably on an adrenaline rush from having such a beautiful baby. You will tire easily. You'll need all of your strength when your little darling decides that two in the morning is playtime, then gets a bellyache at three and is hungry again at four.

Accept any and all offers from your friends and family to baby-sit for an hour here or there so that you can allow your body to get the rest it needs. Let your partner take over for a while. Use baby's naptime for your own naptime. Your body will thank you, because what it needs most right now is rest.

99.

Give Your Body Time to Adjust

"I had the baby. It's been two weeks. I'm still bleeding. I still ache. And why do I still have this darn pregnancy weight on me?"

Over the next few weeks, it will be amazing how quickly your body heals and how fast you actually drop your "baby weight." Within a couple of short months, you will likely be wearing your (looser) pre-pregnancy clothes.

However, after nine months of waiting to get your own body back, you may be anxious to get past all of the discomfort and slink into your old blue jeans. Sorry. Remember that it did take you nine months to get this way. Just because the baby is now on the outside doesn't mean that your body is finished with the whole gestation process.

Give your body the time it needs to repair itself. It will. You'll be good as new in no time—well, in just a little time—although it should be noted that your body will never actually be the same. Your feet will stay a good size larger. Your breasts—after you are finished breastfeeding—may be a size smaller. You may find yourself doing your Kegel exercises religiously to get control of your post-pregnancy bladder.

Aside from that, you will one day look and feel as good as you did before conception. In fact, you'll look even better, because you'll have the satisfaction of motherhood that glows on women's faces. It will just take time. Some mothers claim that it took months after birth to get their bodies back. Others state that it took a year or two before they felt like themselves again. In any case, it will happen.

One day—in a couple of months or years—you will wake up, look in the mirror, and recognize yourself again. Then you'll think, "Wow. That was quick."

100.
Make Every Moment Count

In general, you will feel euphoric every time you look at the newest member of your family. Who can resist playing with a new baby's fingers, taking deep breaths of the sweet-smelling skin, or repeatedly patting the rounded bottom? This is especially true when it's your baby. You will be under a spell even greater than when you fell in love with your mate. In fact, both of you will find yourselves spending hours on end just watching the baby sleep.

What makes this time even more magical is the fact that you will naturally cocoon for a few days or weeks after you bring your baby home. Neither of you will want to be anywhere other than with your baby—and each other. For a while, you will lock the door and let only a few of your closest loved ones into your company. You might not even want to let anyone in, and that's okay, too. The three of you need some quality time to get to know each other right now.

Cocooning after birth is akin to nesting before birth—you are instinctively adjusting to your new life. Besides that, you are probably too tired to go anywhere—but who would want to? You have everything that you've always wanted and needed right in front of you.

Furthermore, there will be a moment a few days after you've brought your newborn home when you will feel total and complete joy. Perhaps you will awaken one morning, look over at the angelic face of the baby asleep in the bassinet next to you, and turn the other way to see your doting husband asleep on your pillow, and it will strike. You will feel deeply and profoundly moved by the miracle of this triangle—your family.

It is a powerful moment when you realize that the love you have for another human being (your mate) has taken shape in the form of your child. When this feeling overtakes you, and it will, it may be one of the happiest moments of your life.

Savor the moment. Take a deep breath and a mental snapshot of the feeling to keep with you forever. On those darker nights, when you need a hug, you'll always have this moment—this feeling of utter love and serenity—to see you through. Good luck.